Second Edition

Y0-BZE-566

Use and
Interpretation of
Tests in
Allergy & Immunology

James B. Peter, M.D., Ph.D.
Ronald A. Blum, Ph.D

Editors

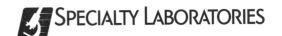

SPECIALTY LABORATORIES

Use and Interpretation of Tests
in Allergy & Immunology

James B. Peter, M.D., Ph.D.
Ronald A. Blum, Ph.D.
Editors

Second Edition - February, 1997

Copyright © Specialty Laboratories
All rights reserved
ISBN 1-889342-06-8

Printed in the United States of America

Specialty Laboratories
2211 Michigan Avenue
Santa Monica, CA 90404-3900
800/421-4449

Dear Colleagues:

In keeping with Specialty Laboratories' core purpose, "We Help Doctors Help Patients", as well as our covenants to provide clinically useful information about cost-effective, leading-edge analyses, the Team of Scientists at *Specialty* are delighted to provide you with this Second Edition of **USE and INTERPRETATION of TESTS in ALLERGY & IMMUNOLOGY**.

The explosive growth of our knowledge of allergy and immunology is paralleled by its clinical application. Data reviewed in this book thoroughly validate the clinical utility of specialized testing not only for diagnosis and prognosis but also for therapeutic monitoring of patients with asthmatic and allergic diseases. As newer and more focused therapies become available, the need for innovative and clinically incisive testing will greatly increase.

To all those charged with the care of patients with asthmatic and allergic disease, this book and our ongoing research are manifestations of our commitment to assist you in these challenging endeavors. We look forward to hearing how subsequent editions of this volume can be made ever more useful.

Sincerely,

The Editors

Dedication And Acknowledgments

The *Specialty* "Orange Book" is dedicated to all who through diligence and painstaking attention to detail advance the frontiers of scientific knowledge. Members of the Research, Development and Clinical Laboratory Teams at Specialty Laboratories are carefully selected for superb technical skills, unwavering commitment to scientific principles and ability to participate in and contribute to *Specialty's* lively intellectual environment. This booklet is our contribution to the challenging task of keeping up with the exciting advances in the study and treatment of allergy and asthma.

The research and support staffs of *Specialty* were instrumental in aiding the ongoing review of literature and synthesis of ideas that make updating and producing a book of this nature possible. Production of the Second Edition of the *Specialty* Orange Book would not have been accomplished without the learned contributions to the content and editing made by the scientists at *Specialty* who wrote and/or updated individual sections of the book. The editors gratefully acknowledge the insightful contributions to the content and organization made by Herminio R. Reyes, Ph.D., the splendid pre-production coordination and document processing assistance of Rose Yesowitch, B.S. and the talented library support of Paul Lomax, R.EEG T. and Carla Herrin, B.A.

Preface

All those who participate in the care of patients with allergic and asthmatic diseases know how explosively these fields are changing. This book is intended as a guide to the incisive use and interpretation of the many techniques now available for the detection of analytes useful in the evaluation of patients with allergic and asthmatic diseases.

For ease of reference, the *Specialty* Orange Book is organized into chapters encompassing:

Evaluation of Allergy • **Evaluation of Humoral Immunity** • **Evaluation of Cellular Immunity** • **Bacterial and Fungal Hypersensitivity Reactions** • **Other Allergic States and Sensitivities** • **Evaluation of Inflammation** • **Evaluation of Complement** • **Viral Infections Associated with Allergy, Asthma and Immunodeficiency States** • **The Neuroimmune Axis**

Brief descriptions of **Receiver Operating Characteristic Curves, Sensitivity, Specificity, and Predictive Values, Methodologies,** tables of **Allergens Which Stimulate T cells, Clusters of Differentiation, Commonly Available Precipitin** and **RAST Tests, Effector Functions of T_H1 and T_H2 $CD4^+$ T-cell Subsets,** and a list of **Abbreviations** are appended. An **Index** lists diseases, organisms and analytes mentioned in the text.

For your convenience, all of our "Use and Interpretation of Tests" books as well as our DIRECTORY OF SERVICES are available on the internet. Be sure to visit our website at: **http://www.specialtylabs.com.**

A tear-out card at the back of this text lists additional publications and resources available from Specialty Laboratories. Please fill out the card if you would like to receive copies of other *Specialty* publications or would like to be placed on our mailing list.

USE AND INTERPRETATION OF TESTS IN ALLERGY & IMMUNOLOGY is designed as an EDUCATIONAL and REFERENCE tool. For information on the availability of specific tests, please contact our Client Services department at 800-421-4449.

Specialty Laboratories
P.O. Box 92722
Los Angeles, CA 90009-9920

Table Of Contents

Chapter 1
Evaluation of Allergy

IgE and IgE Antibodies

Alaa E. Ahmed, Ph.D.

IgE constitutes a fraction of the total antibody in serum (50–300 ng/mL compared to 10 mg/mL for IgG),[1] and together with its Fc receptor (FcεRII), is important in primary immune responses.[2] The immunogenetic mechanisms underlying IgE responsiveness seen in the atopic diseases can be divided into antigen-specific and non-antigen-specific responses. The former is strongly influenced by HLA-D-encoded, MHC class II genes and involves T- and B-cell interactions. The latter, noncognate regulation of IgE, may primarily involve basophils and mast cells, with supplemental involvement of T cells.[2] T-cell activation leads to secretion of IL-4, which provides the first signal for IgE induction and expression of CD40 ligand essential for T-cell induction of IgE.[3] IgE antibodies to common antigens are reported in the serum of 13% of normal blood donors.[4] Autoantibodies to the IgE FcεRII (high affinity receptors) reported in the sera of patients with chronic urticaria, can induce histamine release from mast cells.[5]

REFERENCES

1. Sutton BJ, Gould HJ. The human IgE network. Nature 1993;366:421-8.
2. Marsh DG, Neely JD, Breazeale DR, et al. Linkage analysis of IL4 and other chromosome 5q31.1 markers and total serum immunoglobulin E concentrations. Science 1994;264:1152-6.
3. Vercelli D. Molecular regulation of the IgE immune response. Clin Exp Allergy 1995;25:S2:43-5.
4. Stern A, van Hage-Hamsten M, Sondell K, Johansson SGO. Is allergy screening of blood donors necessary? Vox Sang 1995;69:114-9.
5. Hide M, Francis DM, Grattan CEH, Hakimi J, Kochan JP, Greaves MW. Autoantibodies against the high-affinity IgE receptor as a cause of histamine release in chronic urticaria. N Engl J Med 1993;328:1599-1604.

IgE-Based Assays: See Chapter 4: Alternaria spp., Aspergillus spp. and Cladosporium spp.

IgE Immune Complexes

Alaa E. Ahmed, Ph.D.

In many atopic diseases such as asthma, allergic rhinitis, atopic dermatitis, and hay fever as well as patients with hyper-IgE syndrome and allergic arthralgia, as much as 50% of circulating IgE can be complexed as IgE-IgE or IgE-IgG immune complexes.[1,2] The presence of IgE immune complexes can interfere with assays of serum IgE.[3] In patients with atopic dermatitis, total IgE concentration correlates positively with IgE-IgE immune complexes.[4] Whether these complexes play a role in atopic disease pathophysiology or allergy is unknown.[1-4]

REFERENCES

1. Carini C, Fratazzi C, Barbato M. IgG autoantibody to IgE in atopic patients. Ann Allergy 1988;60:48-52.
2. Boulda L, Berrens L. Do IgE-IgG complexes occur in the circulation. Clin Exp Immunol 1995;100:145-50.
3. Vassella CC, de Weck AL, Stadler BM. Natural anti-IgE auto-antibodies may interfere with diagnostic IgE determination. Clin Exp Immunol 1990;20:295-303.
4. Czech W, Stadler BM, Schopf E, Kapp A. IgE autoantibodies in atopic dermatitis: occurrence of different antibodies against the CH3 and the CH4 epitopes of IgE. Allergy 1995;50:243-8.

Radioallergsorbent Testing (RAST)

Alaa E. Ahmed, Ph.D.

Testing for allergen-specific IgE is useful when skin testing is unreliable due to generalized dermatitis or severe dermatographism, or when the patient is unable to discontinue antihistamines.[1] A significant association is reported between the presence of allergen-specific IgE and a positive skin test.[2] Use of allergenic extracts in skin tests make the comparison between RAST and skin tests difficult due to allergen-dependent and patient-dependent factors, such as the potency of the allergen, number and location of the IgE-binding epitopes on the allergen, number of mast cells and the sensitivity for histamines.[3] Fadal-Nalebuff modified RAST is said to be more sensitive compared to the initial Phadebas RAST and correlates closely with skin testing when skin end point titration is used.[4] Several recombinant allergens are available for both skin tests and RAST.[4-7] Assays for allergen-specific IgG4 are useful largely in patients undergoing desensitization to hymenoptera.[7] Detection of IgG4 antibodies to foods is of no proven diagnostic value.[1]

REFERENCES
1. Smith TF. Allergy testing in clinical practice. Ann Allergy 1992;68:293-301.
2. Dreborg S, Frew A. Allergen standaridization and skin tests. Allergy 1992;14S:49-82.
3. Witteman AM, Stapel SO, Perdok GJ, et al. The relationship between RAST and skin tests results in patients with asthma or rhinitis: A quantitative study with purified major allergens. J Allergy Clin Immunol 1996;97:16-25.
4. Tandy JR, Mabry RL, Mabry CS. Correlation of modified radioallergosorbent test scores and skin test results. Otolaryngol Head Neck Surg 1996;115:42-5.
5. Corey JP, Gungor A. In vitro testing for immunoglobulin E-mediated food allergies. Otolaryngol Head Neck Surg 1996;115:312-8.
6. Menz G, Dolecelk C, Schonheilt-Kenn U, et al. Serological and skin-test diagnosis of birch pollen allergy with recombinant Bet v I, the major birch pollen allergen. Clin Exp Allergy 1996;26:50-60.
7. Watson WT. Food allergy in children. Clin Rev Allergy Immunol 1995;13:347-59.

Skin Testing: See Chapter 5: Delayed-Type Hypersensitivity.

Chapter 2
Evaluation of Humoral Immunity

Chronic and Recurrent Infections

Madhumita Patnaik, M.D.

Antibody immunodeficiency disorders comprise a spectrum of diseases characterized by decreased immunoglobulin levels, ranging from complete absence of all classes of immunoglobulin to selective deficiency of a single class or subclass. There are also cases of specific antibody deficiency, particularly the inability to form antibodies to polysaccharide antigens.[1] Chronic and recurrent infections with encapsulated (polysaccharide-coated) bacteria can be the result of a qualitative deficiency (inability to generate specific antibodies to encapsulated bacteria) or a quantitative deficiency (insufficient levels of immunoglobulins, particularly IgG2), or both qualitative and quantitative deficiencies.[1-3]

EIA for detection of antibodies to polysaccharide antigens of *Streptococcus pneumoniae* types 3, 7F, 9N and 14 is a useful tool for evaluation of humoral immunity.[3] Reports suggest that recurrent infection with *S. pneumoniae* can be a warning sign of immunodeficiency and that patients with multiple myeloma, HIV infection, solid organ tumors and chronic liver disease with bacteremia pneumococcal infections should be offered antipneumococcal vaccines.[4] A fourfold increase in titer of pre- and post-vaccination serum levels of antibodies reactive with diphtheria toxoid, measured by radioantigen binding assay[5] or by EIA, is considered immunologically normal. IgG subclass deficiencies are related to responder/nonresponder status.[6]

Total serum IgG levels are sometimes misleading because serum IgG can be normal in patients with recurrent infections who are IgG2 deficient, but in whom IgG1 and/or IgG3 are elevated.[7] IgG subclass totals by the immunoradiometric assay (IRMA) (IgG1 + IgG2 + IgG3 + IgG4) are much closer to total IgG levels determined by rate nephelometry than are the subclass totals by EIA.[8] See in this Chapter: *Haemophilus influenzae* **b**.

REFERENCES
1. Eibl MM, Wolf HM. Common variable immunodeficiency: clinical aspects and recent progress in identifying the immunological defects. Folia Microbiol (Praha) 1995;40:630-6.
2. Stiehm ER. New and old immunodeficiencies. Pediatr Res 1993;33(Suppl):S2.
3. Boctor FN, Barka NE, Agopian MS. Quantitation of IgG antibody to *Streptococcus pneumoniae* vaccine by ELISA and FAST-ELISA using tyraminated antigen. J Immunol Methods 1989;120:167-71.
4. Rodriguez-Creixems M, Munoz P, Miranda E, et al. Recurrent pneumococcal bacteremia: A warning of immunodeficiency. Arch Intern Med 1996;156:1429-34.
5. Menser MA, Hudson JR. Population studies of diphtheria immunity using antitoxin radioimmunoassay. J Hyg (Lond) 1984;92:1-7.
6. Insel R. Interpreting vaccine responses. In: Wasserman RL, editor. Antibody deficiency: IgG subclass deficiency and vaccine nonresponder states (transcript of a roundtable discussion). Pediatr Infect Dis J 1990;9:424-33.
7. Jefferis R, Kumararatne DS. Selective IgG subclass deficiency: quantification and clinical relevance. Clin Exp Immunol 1990;81:357-67.
8. Agopian M, Peter JB. Comparison of IRMA and EIA in determining IgG subclasses. Unpublished observations, 1990.

Haemophilus influenzae b

Noori E. Barka, Ph.D.

Quantitation of antibodies specific to *H. influenzae* type b (Hib) polyribosyl-ribitolphosphate (PRP) by EIA is the method of choice for assessing the immune status and response to Hib-PRP vaccine.[1,2] EIA allows the detection of Hib IgG-specific antibodies, the predominant isotype for protection against Hib infection.[3] Radioactive antigen binding assay (RABA), the traditional method for detection of Hib antibodies, requires preparation of radioactive antigen; RABA is labor intensive and does not provide quantitation of isotype or subclass-specific antibodies.[2] The concentration of antibodies sufficient to confer protection against Hib is estimated to range from 0.15 to 1 μg antibody protein/mL.[4] A concentration of >0.15 μg/mL can be sufficient to protect unvaccinated individuals while a concentration of >1 μg/mL is considered protective in vaccinated individuals.[5,6] Recurrent Hib infection can occur in many children with Hib antibodies above the protective concentration (1 μg/mL) after vaccination,[7,8] suggesting quantitative assessment of antibodies by itself is insufficient to predict vaccine efficacy and that assessment of antibody avidity and functional capacity should also be used for evaluation of patients with recurrent infection.[4,7,8]

Immunization with PRP conjugate vaccine in which the capsular polysaccharide is covalently linked to proteins such as *N. meningitidis* outer membrane (PRP-OMP), tetanus toxoid (PRP-TT) and diphtheria (PRP-D) is immunogenic, safe and well-tolerated even in infants 2 months of age.[9,10] Vaccination studies in infants show that Hib antibodies can persist for up to 5 years after vaccination with PRP-OMP vaccine.[11] Failure to respond to conjugate vaccination suggests immunodeficiency.[12] With LA (the method of choice), CoA or CIE, Hib antigen can be detected in CSF, serum or urine of most patients with Hib meningitis.[13,14] Detection by EIA can be 16-32 times more analytically sensitive than CoA.[15] Antigen detection is particularly useful when the patient is pretreated with antibiotics. Antigenuria can follow immunization with some Hib conjugate vaccines.[16] Urinary antigen detection tests are unreliable for up to 30 days following vaccination with some conjugate vaccines.[17] Detection of bacteria in CSF by FA staining of membrane filters has good analytical sensitivity, but data on diagnostic sensitivity, specificity and predictive values are not available.[18] Daily serum C-reactive protein (CRP) can be used to monitor children treated for Hib meningitis;[19] CRP becomes normal in children who recover uneventfully in one week but increases after an initial decrease in children with neurologic complications. See in this Chapter: *Streptococcus pneumoniae*.

REFERENCES
1. Phipps DC, Wet J, Eby R, Koster M, Madore DV, Quataert SA. An ELISA employing a *Haemophilus influenzae* type b oligosaccharide-human serum albumin conjugate correlates with the radioantigen binding assay. J Immunol Methods 1990;135:121-8.
2. Madore DV, Anderson P, Baxter BD, et al. Interlaboratory study evaluating quantitation of antibodies to *Haemophilus influenza* type b polysaccharide by enzyme-linked immunosorbent assay. Clin Diagn Lab Immunol 1996;3:84-8.
3. Barra A, Schulz D, Aucouturier P, Preud'homme JL. Measurement of anti-Haemophilus influenzae type b capsular polysaccharide antibodies by ELISA. J Immunol Methods 1988;115:111-7.
4. Granoff DM, Lucas AH. Laboratory correlates of protection against *Haemophilus influenzae* type b disease. Importance of assessment of antibody avidity and immunologic memory. Ann N Y Acad Sci 1995;754:278-88.
5. Käythy H, Peltola H, Karanko V, Mäkelä H. The protective level of serum antibodies to capsular polysaccharide of *Haemophilus influenzae* type b. J Infect Dis 1983;147:1100.
6. Booy R, Hodgson S, Griffiths H, Chapel HM, Moxon ER. Antibody persistence after accelerated immunisation against *Haemophilus influenzae* type b. Br Med J 1993;306:971-2.
7. Ojo-Amaize EA, Church JA, Barka NE, Agopian MS, Peter JB. A rapid and sensitive chemiluminescence assay for evaluation of functional opsonic activity of *Haemophilus influenzae* type b-specific antibodies. Clin Diagn Lab Immunol 1995;2:286-90.
8. Schlesinger Y, Granoff DM, Vaccine Study Group. Avidity and bacterial activity of antibody elicited by different *Haemophilus influenzae* type b conjugate vaccines. JAMA 1992;267:1489-94.
9. Gold R, Scheifele D, Barreto L, et al. Safety and immunogenicity of *Haemophilus influenzae* vaccine (tetanus toxoid conjugate) administered concurrently or combined with diphtheria and tetanus toxoids, pertussis vaccine and inactivated poliomyelitis vaccine to healthy infants at two, four and six months of age. Pediatr Infect Dis J 1994;13:348-55.
10. Kurikka S, Käyhty H, Peltola H, Saarinen L, Eskola J, Mäkelä PH. Neonatal immunization: response to *Haemophilus influenzae* type b-tetanus toxoid conjugate vaccine. Pediatrics 1995;95:815-22.
11. Walter EB, Simmons SS, Clements DA. Anti-polyribosylribitol phosphate antibody levels 5 years after a primary series of *Haemophilus influenzae* type b conjugate vaccine [Letter]. J Infect Dis 1994;170:1050-1.
12. Holmes SJ, Lucas AH, Osterholm MT, Froeschle JE, Granoff DM, The Collaborative Study Group. Immunoglobulin deficiency and idiotype expression in children developing *Haemophilus influenzae* type b disease after vaccination with conjugate vaccine. JAMA 1991;266:1960-5.

13. Burans JP, Tayeb MEL, Abu-Elyazeed R, Woody JN. Comparison of latex agglutination with established bacteriological tests for diagnosis of cerebrospinal meningitis [Letter]. Lancet 1989;2:158-9.
14. Girgis NI, Farid Z, Kilpatrick ME. Diagnosis of bacterial meningitis [Letter]. Lancet 1989;2:1039.
15. Salih MA, Ahmed HS, Hofvander Y, Danielsson D, Olcen P. Rapid diagnosis of bacterial meningitis by an enzyme immunoassay of cerebrospinal fluid. Epidemiol Infect 1989;103:301-10.
16. Rothstein EP, Madore DV, Girone JA, et al. Comparison of antigenuria after immunization with three *Haemophilus influenzae* type b conjugate vaccines. Pediatr Infect Dis J 1991;10:311-4.
17. Goepp JG, Hohenbroken M, Almeido-Hill J, Santosham M. Persistent urinary antigen excretion in infants vaccinated with *Haemophilus influenzae* type b capsular polysaccharide conjugated with outer membrane protein from *Neisseria meningitidis*. Pediatr Infect Dis J 1992;11:2-5.
18. Lim LCL, Pennell DR, Schell RF. Rapid detection of bacteria in cerebrospinal fluid by immunofluorescence staining on membrane filters. J Clin Microbiol 1990;28:670-5.
19. Anttila M, Peltola H. Serum C-reactive protein in the course of *Haemophilus influenzae* type b meningitis. J Infect Dis 1992;165(Suppl 1):S36-7.

IgA Deficiency

Alaa E. Ahmed, Ph.D.

Selective IgA deficiency (IgA-D) is the most common primary immunodeficiency in Caucasian populations, and occurs with a frequency of 1:700 to 1:1600.[1] In IgA-D, patients present with normal IgG and IgM and normal cell-mediated immunity, but are deficient in serum IgA (5 mg/dL as the upper limit for diagnosis).[1] Patients with IgA-D, although asymptomatic, do have an increased frequency of allergies, autoimmune diseases, gastrointestinal disorders, malignancies, ataxia-telangiectasia and congenital rubella.[2] High susceptibility to respiratory tract infection encountered in IgA-D patients is almost always associated with concomitant IgG2 deficiency.[2] IgA-D complicated by a lack of anti-polysaccharide antibodies of the IgG2 subclass or deficiency of serum IgG2, IgG4 and IgE is recognized.[1] The defect in IgA-D is manifested at the stem cell level and bone marrow transfered from an IgA-D donor to a normal recipient results in an IgA-D in the recipient.[1] Some families with IgA-D have first-degree relatives with common variable immunodeficiency (CVID), suggesting that both disorders represent the spectrum of a single disease.[1,2] IgA-D is commonly inherited with an extended haplotype which includes A1, B8 and DR3.[1,4]

CVID affects 1:10,000 individuals. The affected patients are deficient in both IgG and IgA, and in about half of the cases IgM will also be reduced.[1,3] The disorder is usually manifested in teens and can appear in previously healthy individuals.[4] In 12 out of 69 families with IgA-D or CVID, IgA-D and CVID co-occurred; CVID is typically presenting mainly in the parental generation and IgA-D in the children[1]. The nature of the underlying defect in CVID and IgA-D is still unknown.[1,4]

IgA-D is occasionally associated with anti-rheumatic and anti-epileptic therapy including phenytoin, sulfasalazine, penicillamine and captopril.[1] In half of the patients, the deficiency is reversible with cessation of therapy, whereas the remaining patients continue to be deficient.[1] Drug-associated combined deficiency of IgG2 and IgA or CVID can occur.[1,3] Celiac disease is the most common noninfectious intestinal disorder in IgA-D (frequency ~30%).[5] IgA autoantibodies are a common feature in IgA-D (up to 63%).[6,7]

REFERENCES
1. Truedsson L, Baskin B, Pan Q, et al. Genetics of IgA deficiency. APMIS 1995;103:833-42.
2. Espanol T, Catala M, Hernandez M, et al. Development of a common variable immunodeficiency in IgA-deficient patients. Clin Immunol Immunopathol 1996;80:333-5.
3. Ashman RF, Schaffer FM, Kemp JD, et al. Genetic and immunologic analysis of a family containing five patients with common-variable immune deficiency or selective IgA deficiency. J Clin Immunol 1992;12:406-14.
4. Vorechovsky I, Zetterquist H, Paganelli R, et al. The PAX5 gene: a linkage and mutation analysis in candidate human primary immunodeficiencies. Immunogenetics 1995;42:149-52.

5. Meini A, Pillan NM, Villanacci V, et al. Prevalence and diagnosis of celiac disease in IgA-deficient children . Ann Allergy Asthma Immunol 1996;77:333-6.
6. Cunningham-Rundles C. IgA autoantibodies. In: Peter JB, Shoenfeld Y, editors. Autoantibodies. Amsterdam: Elsevier Science B.V., 1996:417-21.
7. Barka NE, Shen GQ, Alosachie IJ, Gershwin ME, Reyes H, Peter JB. Multireactive pattern of serum autoantibodies in asymptomatic individuals with immunoglobulin A deficiency. Clin Diagn Lab Immunol 1995;2:469-72.

IgG Subclasses

Alaa E. Ahmed, Ph.D.

Selective deficiencies of one or more IgG subclasses are associated with sinusitis, recurrent otitis media and/or asthma, recurrent respiratory tract infections with or without IgA deficiency (IgA-D), chronic chest symptoms in nonallergic children, recurrent meningococcemia, recurrent pneumococcal bacteremia, unusual allergies and failure to respond to polysaccharide antigens of certain encapsulated bacteria.[1] In serum, the proportions of IgG subclasses are 60%, 31%, 6% and 3% for IgG1, IgG2, IgG3, and IgG4, respectively.[2] A normal level of total IgG in serum does not rule out a clinically important deficiency of one or more IgG subclasses, due to compensatory increases of other IgG subclasses. Indeed, serum and salivary IgG concentrations are usually within the normal range in idividuals with homozygous gene deletions of either G1, or G4, or both G2 and G4.[1] The constant region of the heavy chains is encoded by one of the immunoglobulin heavy chain genes (CH) localized on chromosome 14.[2] Six different extensive multigene deletions are described in the immunoglobulin CH locus.[2]

Families of individuals with IgA-D should have at least one evaluation of their IgG subclasses because of the close association of IgA-D and variable common immune deficiency (CVID).[3] CVID affects 1:10,000 individuals with a deficiency in both IgG and IgA, and in about half of those patients, IgM will also be reduced.[3] The disorder usually manifests in the teens and can appear in previously healthy individuals.[4] The nature of the underlying defect in CVID and IgA-D is still unknown.[3,4] Preferential active transplacental transport of IgG subclasses is in the order of IgG1, IgG3, IgG2 and IgG4, with levels of IgG changing during the first months of life, depending on both the period of gestation and the infant's postnatal age.[5,6] Some children with IgG2 concentrations 2 SD below the appropriate age-adjusted mean show no evidence of increased susceptibility to infection;[7] quantitative deficiencies of IgG2 or IgG4 or IgG2 and IgG4 do not segregate with high frequency of bacterial infections in HIV-infected children.[8]

Some IgA-deficient patients with normal IgG2 levels and subnormal responses to pneumococcal polysaccharides are susceptible to pneumococcal sepsis.[9] Likewise, invasive *Haemophilus influenzae* b (Hib) disease occurs despite vaccination with Hib-PRP in some children with normal IgG2 levels.[10,11] Although the frequency of failure to respond to polysaccharide antigens is seemingly associated with increased bacterial sepsis,[9] no epidemiologically acceptable data are available to support this. The same is true for the relationship between recurrent bacterial infections and IgG subclass deficiencies. The predictive value of different degrees of deficiency of IgG subclasses for clinical disease (e.g., chronic versus recurrent acute infections) is not established, nor can one reliably predict defects of systemic antibody production based on various degrees of subclass deficiency in young children.[10] Total IgG2 concentrations do correlate, however, with responses to polysaccharide antigens in normal adults.[11]

Quantitation of antigen-specific antibodies among the four subclasses of IgG does not often yield clinically useful information, but lack of adequate standardization of assays for antigen-specific IgG subclasses might obscure important correlations. In general, early immune response to antigens is largely restricted to the IgG1 subclass, regardless of whether exposure is by injection, via the gut, or by inhalation.[11]

Protein antigens characteristically induce antibodies of the IgG1/IgG3 or IgG1/IgG4 subclasses, and, of these, the highest affinity antibodies are IgG1. Polysaccharide antigens characteristically induce antibodies of the IgG2 subclass, with relative avidities IgG2 > IgG1.[13] The clear-cut influence of Gm allotypes on the serum concentrations of IgG1, IgG2, and IgG3 is not yet recognized to be of clinical importance.[14] The cellular and molecular basis for immunoglobulin deficiencies, the clinical features of immunoglobulin deficiency syndromes, and the therapy of immunoglobulin deficiencies are reviewed.[13,15] See in this Chapter: *Haemophilus influenzae* b.

REFERENCES
1. Plebani A, Ugazio G, Meini A, et al. Extensive deletion of immunoglobulin heavy chain constant region genes in the absence of recurrent infections: when is IgG subclass deficiency clinically relevant? Clin Immunol Immunopathol 1993;68:46-51.
2. Engstrom PE, Norhagen G, Osipova EL, et al. Salivary IgG subclasses in individuals with and without homozygous IGHG gene deletions. Immunology 1996;89:178-82.
3. Ashman RF, Schaffer FM, Kemp JD, et al. Genetic and immunologic analysis of a family containing five patients with common-variable immune deficiency or selective IgA deficiency. J Clin Immunol 1992;12:406-14.
4. Vorechovsky I, Zetterquist H, Paganelli R, et al. The PAX5 gene: a linkage and mutation analysis in candidate human primary immunodeficiencies. Immunogenetics 1995;42:149-52.
5. Drossou V, Kanakoudi F, Diamanti E, et al. Concentrations of main serum opsonins in early infancy. Arch Dis Child Fetal Neonatal Ed 1995;72:F172-175.
6. Wilczynski J, Lukasik B. Transplacental transfer of antibodies to some respiratory viruses. Acta Microbiol Pol 1994;43:347-58.
7. Shackelford PG, Granoff DM, Madassery JV, et al. Clinical and immunologic characteristics of healthy children with subnormal serum concentrations of IgG2. Pediatr Res 1990;27:16-21.
8. Roilides E, Black C, Reimer C, Rubin M, Venzon D, Pizzo PA. Serum immunoglobulin G subclasses in children infected with human immunodeficiency virus type I. Pediatr Infect Dis J 1991;10:134-9.
9. Truedsson L, Baskin B, Pan Q, et al. Genetics of IgA deficiency. APMIS 1995;103:833-42.
10. Pertmer TM, Roberts TR, Haynes JR. Influenza virus nucleoprotein-specific immunoglobulin G subclass and cytokine responses elicited by DNA vaccination are dependent on the route of vector DNA delivery. J Virol 1996;70:6119-25.
11. Siber GR, Santosham M, Reid R, et al. Impaired antibody response to Haemophilus influenzae type b polysaccharide and low IgG2 and IgG4 concentrations in Apache children. N Engl J Med 1990;323:1387-92.
12. Peterson TD, Ciofu O, Pressler T, et al. Quantitative analysis of the IgG and IgG subclass immune response to chromosomal pseudomonos aeruginosa beta-lactamase in serum from patients with cystic fibrosis by western blotting and laser scanning densitometry. Thorax 1996;51:733-8.
13. Rosen FS, Cooper MD, Wedgwood RJP. The primary immunodeficiencies. N Eng J Med 1995;333:431-40.
14. Oxelius VA, Eibl MM. Different Gm allotype amounts in human intravenous immunoglobulin (IVIG) preparations; survival of foreign Gm allotypes in immunodeficient patients. Clin Exp Immunol 1996;106:203-7.
15. Huston DP, Kavanaugh AF, Rohane PW, Huston MM. Immunoglobulin deficiency syndromes and therapy. J Allergy Clin Immunol 1991;87:1-17.

Mannan-Binding Protein

Vellalore N. Kakanaiah, Ph.D.

Serum mannan-binding protein (Man-BP), a C-type lectin that binds to mannose and N-acetylglucosamine on viruses or organisms such as Gram-negative bacteria, belongs to a defined subgroup of proteins called collectins,[1] and plays a crucial role in the first line of host defense against these pathogens by functioning as an opsonin.[2-4] Structurally, Man-BP is similar to C1q, a subcomponent of the first complement component which binds to the C1q receptor and activates the complement cascade,[5] leading to the direct killing of bacteria.[6,7] Deficiency of Man-BP is associated with failure to opsonize bakers yeast (*Saccharomyces cerevisiae*), but the high frequency (~5–7%) of impaired opsonic function in normal populations shows that the putative relationship of Man-BP-deficiency to recurrent infections, chronic diarrhea, otitis media or allergies is not straightforward.[8] Man-BP is probably a common risk factor for infection in infants ages 6–24 months,[8] because a frequency of the mutant allele estimated at about 3% would account for a 5–7% frequency of impaired opsonic function.[9] Second (co-existing) partial deficiencies (e.g., both Man-BP and C4 or both Man-BP and an immunoglobulin abnormality) could predispose to infection in a substantial number of individuals at various ages.[10] The mutant allele of Man-BP gene represents a minor risk factor for SLE.[11] *Pneumocystis carinii* is ingested via the mannose receptor of alveolar macrophages.[12]

REFERENCES
1. Holmskov U, Malhotra R, Sim RB, Jensenius JC. Collectins: collagenous C-type lectins of the innate immune defense system. Immunol Today 1994;15:67-74.
2. Summerfield JA. The role of mannose-binding protein in host defense. Biochem Soc Trans 1993;21:473-7.
3. Kuhlman M, Joiner K, Ezekowitz RAB. The human mannose-binding protein functions as opsonin. J Exp Med 1989;169:1733-45.
4. Hartshorn KL, Sastry K, White MR, et al. Human mannose-binding protein functions as an opsonin for influenza A viruses. J Clin Invest 1993;91:1414-20.
5. Ikeda K, Sannoh T, Kawasaki N, Kawasaki T, Yamashina I. Serum lectin with known structure activates complement through the classical pathway. J Biol Chem 1987;262:7451-4.
6. Kawasaki N, Kawasaki T, Yamashina I. A serum lectin (mannan-binding protein) has complement-dependent bactericidal activity. J Biochem 1989;106:483-9.
7. Schweinle JE, Ezekowitz RAB, Tenner A, Kuhlman M, Joiner KA. Human mannose-binding protein activates the alternative complement pathway and serum bactericidal activity on a mannose-rich isolate of Salmonella. J Clin Invest 1989;84:1821-9.
8. Super M, Thiel S, Lu J, et al. Association of low levels of mannan-binding protein with a common defect of opsonisation. Lancet 1989;2:1236-9.
9. Sumiya M, Super M, Tabona P, et al. Molecular basis of opsonic defect in immunodeficient children. Lancet 1991;337:1569-70.
10. Turner MW. Deficiency of mannan binding protein - a new complement deficiency syndrome. Clin Exp Immunol 1991;86:S53-6.
11. Davies EJ, Snowden N, Hillarby MC, et al. Mannose-binding protein gene polymorphism in systemic lupus erythematosus. Arthritis Rheum 1995;38:110-4.
12. Ezekowitz RAB, Williams DJ, Koziel H, et al. Uptake of *Pneumocystis carinii* mediated by the macrophage mannose receptor. Nature 1991;351:155-8.

Opsonophagocytosis

Emmanuel A. Ojo-Amaize, Ph.D.

Serum bactericidal activity and phagocytic killing are two important mechanisms involved in host defense against bacteria.[1] Antibodies and/or complement, especially the third component, serve as opsonins to bind to antigenic determinants on microorganisms and increase their susceptibility to phagocytosis by polymorphonuclear leukocytes, especially neutrophils.[2] The availability of opsonic antimicrobial antibodies is essential for optimal function of phagocytes in uptake and containment of bacteria.[3] Sera of 50% of children with recurrent *Haemophilus influenzae* b (Hib) infection lack opsonophagocytic activity against Hib.[4] IgG opsonins with poor opsononizing capacities in the airway can contribute to the chronic problem of infection, as seen in patients with cystic fibrosis[5] and AIDS.[6] In pneumococcal and Hib infections, phagocytosis is significantly enhanced with both specific IgG1 and IgG2 in the presence of complement. However, in the absence of complement, only IgG2 is an active opsonin.[7] Colony counting, the "gold standard" for assaying killing and phagocytosis of microbes, is replaced by tests such as chemiluminescence[4] and flow cytometry.[8]

REFERENCES
1. Lagergard T, Frish A, Purven M, Nilsson LA. Serum bactericidal activity and phagocytosis in host defense against *Haemophilus ducreyi*. Microb Pathog 1995;18:37-51.
2. Bruyn GAW, Zegers JM, van Furth R. Mechanisms of host defense against infection with *Streptococcus pneumoniae*. Clin Infect Dis 1991;14:251-62.

3. Salvadori LG, Blake MS, McCarty M, et al. Group A streptococcus-liposome ELISA antibody titers to group A polysaccharide and opsonophagocytic capabilities of the antibodies. J Infect Dis 1995;171:593-600.
4. Ojo-Amaize EA, Church JA, Barka NE, et al. A rapid and sensitive chemiluminensce assay for evaluation of functional opsonic activity of *Haemophilus influenzae* type b-specific antibodies. Clin Diagn Lab Immunol 1995;2:286-90.
5. Pier GB. Analysis of naturally occurring antibodies to mucoid *Pseudomonas aeruginosa* in cystic fibrosis patients. J Infect Dis 1996;173:513-5.
6. Kumar PN, Collins MS, Pierce PF. Anti-lipopolysaccharide antibody levels in patients with AIDS at the onset of *Pseudomonas aeruginosa* bacteremia. J Acquir Immun Defic Syndr 1994;7:587-91.
7. Kaniuk ASC, Lortan JE, Monteil MA. Specific IgG subclass antibody levels and phagocytosis of serotype 14 pneumococcus following immunization. Scand J Immunol 1992;36:98-8.
8. Troelstra A, Vogel L, van Alphen L, et al. Opsonic antibodies to outer membrane protein P2 of nonencapsulated *Haemophilus influenzae* are strain specific. Infect Immun 1994;62:779-84.

Streptococcus pneumoniae

James B. Estes, M.A., MT(ASCP)

S. pneumoniae infection is a leading cause of acute respiratory tract infection (pneumonia), with a prevalence of ≤12/1000 of the general population; as well as bacteremia and meningitis, and accounts for approximately 40,000 deaths per year.[1-4] The incidence of pneumococcal infection increases in the elderly and children and is associated with many chronic diseases, including sickle cell disease, endocarditis, liver and kidney diseases, head injury, lymphoproliferative diseases, cerebral hemorrhage, rheumatic fever, otitis media, asthma, obstructive pulmonary diseases, septicemia, diabetes mellitus and Guillain-BarrJ syndrome.[1,2,5-8] Protocols for vaccination using various polysaccharide *S. pneumoniae* antigens are established.[9,10] Criteria for immunization in immunosuppressed patients, including HIV seropositives, are also evaluated.[11,12] Patient age and post-immunization interval are important factors in the evaluation of antibody responses following infection or vaccination. Pediatric pneumonia IgG responses reach a maximum at 12 months and its clinical course is not substantially altered by HIV infection.[13] IgM concentrations increases in children from <4% prevalence at 16 months to 50% at 2 years; while IgA concentrations increase approximately 35-fold in 6–18 months old children 4 weeks after immunization.[14-16] Several other variables were shown to affect the clinical course and antibody response in *S. pneumoniae* infection. Lack of maternal breast feeding and exposure to tobacco are risk factors for acquiring invasive disease.[17] Immunosuppressive conditions such as AIDS, organ transplants and splenectomy have increased the rate of community-acquired pneumonia (CAP).[18-20] Antibody responses to pneumococcal polysaccharides are rated as strong to types 3, 18 and 18C; moderate to types 7F, 9N and 12 and weak to types 1, 6A, 14 and 19 and are predominantly of the IgG2 subclass.[21-23] Antibody responses to other *S. pneumoniae* antigens, such as pneumolysin and PspA have uncertain clinical utility.[24,25]

Impaired responses to *S. pneumoniae* antigens are reported in ataxia-telangiectasia, Wiskott-Aldrich syndrome, vitamin B and complement deficiencies, Sjögren syndrome, chronic chest symptoms and both IgG2 and IgA deficiencies.[26-31] Antibiotic resistant strains are increasing in prevalence with a consequential increase in CAP frequency.[32-35] Screening for antibody responses to *S. pneumoniae* antigens is usually performed by latex agglutination.[36,37] Serotyping and confirmation of infection are accomplished by sensitive EIAs and PCRs. Culture and PCR methods are able to detect non-antigen-producing *S. pneumoniae* colonization.[38-42] See in this Chapter: ***Haemophilus influenzae* b.**

REFERENCES
1. Noah ND. Vaccination against pneumococcal infection. Br Med J 1988;297:1351-2.
2. Mäkelä PH, Jokinen C, PyhäläR, Mäkelä M, Ruutu P. Use of vaccines for respiratory infections. Strategies for influenza and pneumococcal vaccines. Scand J Infect Dis Suppl 1990;70:141-8.

3.   Venkatesan P, Macfarlane JT, Finch RG.   Pneumococcal antigens revisited. Infectious Disease Newsletter 1993;12:5-6.
4.   Bartlett JG, Mundy LM.   Community-acquired pneumonia.   N Engl J Med 1995;333:1618-24.
5.   Swanson JA, Hoecker JL.   Otitis media in young children.   Mayo Clin Proc 1996;71:179-83.
6.   McLaren MJ, Markowitz M, Gerber MA.   Rheumatic heart disease in developing countries: the consequence of inadequate prevention [Editorial].   Ann Intern Med 1994;120:243-5.
7.   Terryberry J, Sutjita M, Shoenfled Y, et al.   Myelin- and microbe-specific antibodies in Guillain-Barré syndrome.   J Clin Lab Anal 1995;9:308-19.
8.   Bruyn GAW, Hiemstra PS, Matze-van der Lans A, van Furth R.   Pneumococcal anticapsular antibodies in patients with chronic cardiovascular and obstructive lung disease in the Netherlands.   J Infect Dis 1990;162:1192-4.
9.   Austrian R.   Pneumococcal polysaccharide vaccines.   Rev Infect 1989;11(Suppl 3):S598-602.
10.   Steinhoff MC, Edwards K, Keyserling H, et al.   A randomized comparison of three bivalent Streptococcus pneumoniae glycoprotein conjugate vaccines in young children: effect of polysaccharide size and linkage characteristics.   Pediatr Infect Dis J 1994;13:368-72.
11.   Jain A, Jain S, Gant V.   Should patients positive for HIV infection receive pneumococcal vaccine?   Br Med J 1995;310:1060-2.
12.   Rodriguez-Barradas MC, Musher DM, Lahart C, et al.   Antibody to capsular polysaccharides of Streptococcus pneumoniae after vaccination of human immunodeficiency virus-infected subjects with 23-valent pneumococcal vaccine.   J Infect Dis 1992;165:553-6.
13.   Gesner M, Desiderio D, Kim M, et al.   Streptococcus pneumoniae in human immunodeficiency virus type 1-infected children.   Pediatr Infect Dis J 1994;13:697-703.
14.   Pomat WS, Smith TA, Sanders RC, et al.   Levels of anti-pneumococcal antibodies in young children in Papua New Guinea.   Epidemiol Infect 1993;111:109-19.
15.   Brhssow H, Baensch M, Sidoti J.   Seroprevalence of immunoglobulin M (IgM) and IgG antibodies to polysaccharides of Streptococcus pneumoniae in different age groups of Ecuadorian and German children.   J Clin Microbiol 1992;30:2765-71.
16.   Witt CS, Pomat W, Lehmann D, Alpers MP.   Antibodies to pneumococcal polysaccharides in pneumoniae and response to pneumococcal vaccination in young children in Papua New Guinea.   Clin Exp Immunol 1991;83:219-24.
17.   Gessner BD, Ussery XT, Parkinson AJ, Breiman RF.   Risk factors for invasive disease caused by Streptococcus pneumoniae among Alaska native children younger than two years of age.   Pediatr Infect Dis J 1995;14:123-8.
18.   Marrie TJ.   Community-acquired pneumonia.   Clin Infect Dis 1994;18:501-15.
19.   Lortan JE, Vellodi A, Jurges ES, Hugh-Jones K.   Class- and subclass-specific pneumococcal antibody levels and response to immunization after bone marrow transplantation.   Clin Exp Immunol 1992;88:512-9.
20.   Konradsen HB, Nielsen JL, Pedersen FK, Henrichsen J.   Antibody persistence in splenectomized adults after pneumococcal vaccination.   Scand J Infect Dis 1990;22:725-7.
21.   Bardardottir E, Jonsson S, Jonsdottir I, Sigfusson A, Valdimarsson H.   IgG subclass response and opsonization of Streptococcus pneumoniae after vaccination of healthy adults.   J Infect Dis 1990;162:482-8.
22.   Prellner K, Kalm O, Harsten G, Heldrup J, Oxelius V-A.   Pneumococcal serum antibody concentrations during the first three years of life: a study of otitis-prone and non-otitis-prone children.   Int J Pediatr Otorhinolaryngol 1989;17:267-79.
23.   Leinonen M, Sakkinen A, Kalliokoski R, et al.   Antibody response to 14-valent pneumococcal capsular polysaccharide vaccine in pre-school age children.   Pediatr Infect Dis 1986;5:39-44.
24.   Kanclerski K, Blomquist S, Granström M, Möllby R.   Serum antibodies to pneumolysin in patients with pneumonia.   J Clin Microbiol 1988;26:96-100.
25.   Crain MJ, Waltman WD II, Turner JS, et al.   Pneumococcal surface protein A (PspA) is serologically highly variable and is expressed by all clinically important capsular serotypes of Streptococcus pneumoniae.   Infect Immun 1990;58:3293-9.
26.   Fata FT, Herzlich BC, Schiffman G, Ast AL.   Impaired antibody responses to pneumococcal polysaccharide in elderly patients with low serum vitamin B_{12} levels.   Ann Intern Med 1996;124:299-304.
27.   Herer B, Labrousse F, Mordelet-Dambrine M, et al.   Selective IgG subclass deficiencies and antibody responses to pneumococcal capsular polysaccharide antigen in adult community-acquired pneumonia.   Am Rev Respir Dis 1990;142:854-7.
28.   French MAH, Denis KA, Dawkins R, Peter JB.   Severity of infections in IgA deficiency: correlation with decreased serum antibodies to pneumococcal polysaccharides and decreased serum IgG2 and/or IgG4.   Clin Exp Immunol 1995;100:47-53.
29.   Ambrosino DM, Siber GR, Chilmonczyk BA, Jernberg JB, Finberg RW.   An immunodeficiency characterized by impaired antibody responses to polysacchardies.   N Engl J Med 1987;316:790-3.

30. Bruyn GAW, Hiemstra PS, Rijkers GT. Type-specific anti-pneumococcal antibodies in a vaccinated patient with combined immunoglobulin A and IgG2 deficiency and invasive pneumococcal infections [Letter]. J Infect Dis 1992;166:1460-1.
31. Hazlewood MA, Kumararatne DS, Webster ADB, Goodall M, Bird P, Daha M. An association between homozygous C3 deficiency and low levels of anti-pneumococcal capsular polysaccharide antibodies. Clin Exp Immunol 1992;87:404-9.
32. MuZoz R, Coffey TJ, Daniels M, et al. Intercontinental spread of a multiresistant clone of serotype 23F *Streptococcus pneumoniae*. J Infect Dis 1991;164:302-6.
33. Jernigan DB, Cetron MS, Breiman RF. Minimizing the impact of drug-resistant *Streptococcus pneumoniae* (DRSP). JAMA 1996;275:206-9.
34. Breiman RF, Butler JC, Tenover FC, Elliott JA, Facklam RR. Emergence of drug-resistant pneumococcal infections in the United States. JAMA 1994;271:1831-5.
35. Friedland IR, McCracken GH Jr. Management of infections caused by antibiotic-resistant *Streptococcus pneumoniae*. N Engl J Med 1994;331:377-82.
36. Witt CS, Montgomery JM, Pomat W, Lehmann D, Alpers MP. Detection of *Streptococcus pneumoniae* and *Haemophilus influenzae* type b antigens in the serum and urine of patients with pneumonia in Papua New Guinea: comparison of latex agglutination and counterimmunoelectrophoresis. Rev Infect Dis 1990;12(Suppl 8):S1001-5.
37. Holloway Y, Boersma WG, Kuttschrhtter H, Snijder JAM. Minimum number of pneumococci required for capsular antigen to be detectable by latex agglutination. J Clin Microbiol 1992;30:517-38.
38. Boersma WG, Lòwenberg A, Holloway Y, Kuttschrhtter H, Snijder JAM, KoNter H. The role of antigen detection in pneumococcal carriers: a comparison between cultures and capsular antigen detection in upper respiratory tract secretions. Scand J Infect Dis 1993;25:51-6.
39. Boctor FN, Barka NE, Agopian MS. Quantitation of IgG antibody to *Streptococcus pnuemoniae* vaccine by ELISA and FAST-ELISA using tyraminated antigen. J Immunol Methods 1989;120:167-71.
40. Zhang Y, Isaacman DJ, Wadowsky RM, Rydquist-White J, Post JC, Ehrlich GD. Detection of *Streptococcus pneumoniae* in whole blood by PCR. J Clin Microbiol 1995;33:596-601.
41. Gillespie SH, Ullman C, Smith MD, Emery V. Detection of *Streptococcus pneumoniae* in sputum samples by PCR. J Clin Microbiol 1994;32:1308-11.
42. Rådström P, Bäckman A, Qian N, Kragsbjerg P, Påhlson C, Olcén P. Detection of bacterial DNA in cerebrospinal fluid by an assay for simultaneous detection of *Neisseria meningitidis*, *Haemophilus influenzae*, and streptococci using a seminested PCR strategy. J Clin Microbiol 1994;32:2738-44.

Chapter 3
Evaluation of Cellular Immunity

Beta Thromboglobulin

Alaa E. Ahmed, Ph.D.

Beta thromboglobulin (βTG), a chemokine derived through successive proteolysis of platelet basic protein (PBP), is a 94 amino acid protein found in the alpha granules of platelets.[1] Because βTG is degraded more slowly than platelet factor-4 (PF4), the plasma concentrations of both granule constituents (βTG and PF4) are measured for assessment of platelet activation in allergic states and asthma.[2] Increased ratios of βTG to PF4 (indices of platelet activation) suggest that platelet activation plays a role in exercise-induced[4] and nocturnal asthma,[3] but is not a major contributor to cold urticaria[5] or histamine-induced bronchoconstriction.[2] Elevated βTG concentrations are also found in a variety of diseases associated with platelet activation such as atrial fibrillation and myeloproliferative disorders.[6,7] See in this Chapter: **Platelet Factor 4** and **Neutrophil Activating Peptide 2**.

REFERENCES

1. Amiral J, Maraing-Koka A, Wolf M, et al. Presence of autoantibodies to interleukin-8 or neutrophil-activating peptide-2 in patients with heparin-associated thrombocytopenia. Blood 1996;88:410-6.
2. Oppenheim JJ, Zachariae CC, Mukaida N, Matsushima K. Properties of the novel proinflammatory supergene "intercrine" cytokine family. Annu Rev Immunol 1991;9:617-48.
3. Morrison JF, Pearson SB, Dean HG, Craig IR, Bramley PN. Platelet activation in nocturnal asthma. Thorax 1991;46:197-200.
4. Johnson CE, Belfield PW, Davis S, Cooke NJ, Spencer A, Davies JA. Platelet activation during exercise induced asthma: effect of prophylaxis with cromoglycate and salbutamol. Thorax 1986;41:290-4.
5. Ormerod AD, Kobza Black A, Dawes J, et al. Prostaglandin D2 and histamine release in cold urticaria unaccompanied by evidence of platelet activation. J Allergy Clin Immunol 1988;82:586-9.
6. Lip GYH, LIP PL, Zarifis J, et al. Fibrin D-Dimer and β-thromboglobulin as markers of thrombogenesis and platelet activation in atrial fibrilation. Circulation 1996;94:425-31.
7. Fabris F, Luzzatto G, Randi ML, et al. Beta-thromboglobulin and platelet factor-4 in patients with myeloproliferative diseases. Thromb Haemost 1994;72:484-5.

Chemotactic Disorders

E. Robert Wassman, M.D.

Chemotactic disorders are due to various abnormalities of the complex cascade involved with mobilizing an appropriate phagocytic cell response to injury or inflammation. Quantitative or qualitative defects of either the humoral or cellular components of chemotaxis are encountered in a wide variety of clinical settings and generally result in recurrent infections.[1] The overall chemotactic process involves initial generation of chemoattractants, perhaps by local endothelial cells. Common chemoattractants which are important *in vivo* are the anaphylatoxins (C3a, C4a and C5a), leukotriene B_4 (LTB$_4$), IL-8, GM-CSF and platelet-activating factor. Circulating neutrophils, exposed to such chemoattractants, begin a four stage process of emigration through the endothelial barrier to the site of tissue injury where phagocytosis occurs. The four stages of this process are dependent upon the up- and down-regulation of distinct adhesion factors: 1) rolling or initial margination by the selectins (L-, P-, E-); 2) stopping on the endothelium by CD18 integrins and ICAM-1; 3) neutrophil-neutrophil adhesion by CD11b/CD18; and 4) transendothelial migration by CD11b/CD18, CD11a/CD18, ICAM-1.[1] Defects in chemotaxis can be acquired or inherited. An inherited deficiency of the β2 integrins (CD18) results in leukocyte adhesion deficiency in humans and animals which lack p150,95 glycoproteins on leukocytes. This is referred to as "Mac-1," "LFA-1," "Mo-1," "Leu-CAM" or "CR3" deficiencies. Skin windows or biopsies devoid of neutrophils in the face of 5-20 fold peripheral blood leukocytosis is characteristic. The severity of the phenotype varies with the degree of CD18 deficiency which can be demonstrated by flow cytometry. Various mutations in this gene can be demonstrated by molecular analysis and correlated with the severity. Allogeneic bone marrow transplantation is successful and gene therapy of stem cells is promising.[1]

Neonatal neutrophils also show defective adhesion as do neutrophils in patients with specific granule deficiencies (genetic or myeloproliferative conditions). Defects in glycosylation of the critical molecules can also cause chemotactic disorders, as with the Rambon-Hasharon syndrome. The cellular mechanism of observed chemotactic abnormalities are less well defined in Kartagener syndrome (abnormal microtubules), Chediak-Higashi syndrome (giant dysfunctional granules), myeloproliferative disorders (granule defects, decreased deformability or deletion in the chromosome region 7q21-q22 encoding a neutrophil migration factor), storage disorders (type 1b glycogen storage disease, mannosidois), Schwachman-Diamond syndrome, localized juvenile periodontitis (chemotactic factor receptors) and hyperimmunoglobulin E- "Job" syndrome (relative deficiency of IFN-γ).[1,2] Unclassified chemotactic disorders are associated with acute inflammation, viral and bacterial infections, neoplasia (leukemia, Hodgkin disease, Sezary syndrome) and autoimmune disorders (SLE, RA, HIE, diabetes, glomerulonephritis). Recently, it appears that excesses of the chemotactic cascade may underly a variety of conditions such as psoriasis (psoriasin),[3] HIV dementia (TGF-β1),[4] and eosinophilic pulmonary infiltrative disorders (RANTES).[5]

Chemotactic defects are frequently overlooked clinically because the profile of recurrent infection is not associated with overt neutropenia. *In vitro* laboratory correlations of abnormal cellular motility have been infrequent and require highly specialized assays, including the Boyden chamber assay, migration under agarose, radioassay for migration of ^{51}Cr-labeled neutrophils and multicell microwell assays, which utilize small samples. Complexities of these assays relate to ambiguities about observed variables (e.g., the distance of migration and/or the number of migrating cells) as well as the need for specialized real-time image analysis systems for measurements. Variations in the laboratory evaluation also derive from the variability among patients, reflecting both underlying genetic variation and the coexistence of acquired chemotactic defects with acute and chronic inflammation.[1,2] See Chapter 6: **C3a, C4a and C5a Anaphylatoxins** and **Platelet-Activating Factor.**

REFERENCES
1. Anderson DC, Kishimoto TK, Smith CW. Leukocyte adhesion deficiency and other disorders of leukocyte adherence and motility. In: Scriver CR, Beaudet AL, Sly WL, Valle D, editors. The metabolic and molecular bases of inherited disease. Seventh Edition. New York: Mc-Graw-Hill, Inc., 1995;3955-94.
2. Kishimoto TK. A dynamic model for neutrophil localization to inflammatory sites. J NIH Res 1991;3:75.
3. Jinquan T, Vorum H, Larsen CG, et al. Psoriasin: a novel chemotactic protein. J Invest Dermatol 1996;107:5-10.
4. Kwon OJ, Jose PJ, Robbins RA, et al. Glucocorticoid inhibition of RANTES expression in human lung epithelial cells. Am J Respir Cell Mol Biol 1995;12:488-96.
5. Rasty S, Thatikunta P, Gordon J, et al. Human immunodeficiency virus tat gene transfer to the murine central nervous system usinga replication-defective herpes simplex virus vector stimulates transforming growth factor beta 1 gene expression. Proc Natl Acad Sci USA 1996;93:6073-8.

Chemotactic Factors

Vellalore N. Kakanaiah, Ph.D.
Accumulation of neutrophils at sites of inflammation requires a series of steps, including directed migration (chemotaxis), which is mediated largely by components of the complement system (C5a and C5a des Arg). Other chemoattractants for neutrophils include products of bacteria (e.g., N-formyl methionyl peptides), products of fibrinolysis, oxidized lipids (e.g., leukotriene B$_4$) and products of stimulated leukocytes. Interleukin 8 (previously known as neutrophil activating peptide 1) was the first chemotactic cytokine discovered which possesses chemotactic activity for PMNS.[1] Currently, chemokines that possess chemotactic activity for PMNs include epithelial cell-derived neutrophil activating peptide (ENA-78), neutrophil activating peptide 2 (NAP-2), growth-related oncogene (GRO-α, β and γ) and macrophage inflammatory protein-2α and β (MIP-2α and β). Other chemokines belonging to this

supergene family (α-chemokine) which are not chemotactic for neutrophils include platelet factor-4 (PF-4), and an interferon-inducible protein (IIP-10). Related polypeptides with chemotactic activity, predominantly for mononuclear cells (β-chemokines), include monocyte chemoattractant protein-1, 2, and 3 (MCP-1, MCP-2, and MCP-3), macrophage inflammatory protein-1 (MIP-1) α and β, and RANTES.[2,3] These β-chemokines (RANTES, MIP-1α, and MIP-1β) play a major role in HIV infection as suppressive factors.[4]

Both inflammatory and noninflammatory cells are sources of these chemotactic factors. Thus, neutrophils, macrophages, smooth muscle cells, fibroblasts, epithelial cells and endothelial cells are a rich source of chemokines, especially IL-8. Neutrophils can generate IL-8 in response to both endogenous and exogenous signals.[2,3]

MCP-1 is involved in the recruitment of monocytes in a variety of pathologic or physiologic conditions,[5] including solid tumors,[6] inflammatory skin disease,[7] malignant fibrous histiocytoma,[8] alveolar epithelium,[9] ocular inflammation[10] and acute renal allograft rejection.[11]

Assays for measuring neutrophil chemotaxis are usually performed by the microchamber technique or the agarose migration technique.[12] The former is the method of choice because of its greater sensitivity.

Chemotactic assays can be used to test for the presence of inhibitors of chemotaxis in the serum, including those observed in Hodgkin disease, Chediak-Higashi syndrome, diabetes mellitus, rheumatoid arthritis, elevated IgE syndromes, chronic granulomatous disease and mucocutaneous candidiasis. See Chapter 6: **Interleukin 8** and **Chemokines.**

REFERENCES
1. Matsushima K, Oppenheim JJ. Interleukin-8 and MCAF: novel inflammatory cytokines inducible by IL-1 and TNF. Cytokine 1990;1:2-13.
2. Miller MD, Krangel MS. Biology and biochemistry of the chemokines: a family of chemotactic and inflammatory cytokines. Crit Rev Immunol 1992;12:17-46.
3. Kunkel SL, Lukacs NW, Strieter RM. The role of interleukin-8 in the infectious process. Ann N Y Acad Sci 1994;730:134-43.
4. Cocchi F, DeVico AL, Garzino-Demo A, Arya SK, Gallo RC, Lusso P. Identification of RANTES, MIP-1α and MIP-1β as the major HIV-suppressive factors produced by CD8$^+$ T cells. Science 1995;270:1811-5.
5. Leonard EJ, Yoshimura T. Human monocyte chemoattractant protein-1 (MCP-1). Immunol Today 1990;11:97-101.
6. Graves DT, Valente AJ. Monocyte chemotactic proteins from human tumor cells. Biochem Pharmacol 1991;41:333-7.
7. Camp RD. Polypeptide neutrophil chemoattractants in the skin. Dermatologica 1989;179(Suppl 1):20-4.
8. Takeya M, Yoshimura T, Leonard EJ, et al. Production of monocyte chemoattractant protein-1 by malignant fibrous histiocytoma: relation to the origin of histiocyte-like cells. Exp Mol Pathol 1991;54:61-71.
9. Standiford TJ, Kunkel SL, Phan SH, et al. Alveolar macrophage-derived cytokines induce monocyte chemoattractant protein-1 expression from human pulmonary type II-like epithelial cells. J Biol Chem 1991;266:9912-8.
10. Elner SG, Strieter RM, Elner VM, et al. Monocyte chemotactic protein gene expression by cytokine-treated human retinal pigment epithelial cells. Lab Invest 1991;64:819-25.
11. Prodjosudjadi W, Daha MR, Gerritsma JS, et al. Increased urinary excretion of monocyte chemoattractant protein-1 during acute renal allograft rejection. Nephrol Dial Transplant 1996;11:1096-103.
12. Van Damme J, Decock B, Bertini R, et al. Production and identification of natural monocyte chemotactic protein from virally infected murine fibroblasts. Relationship with the product of the mouse competence (JE) gene. Eur J Biochem 1991;199:223-9.

Connective Tissue Activating Peptide-III

Herminio R. Reyes, Ph.D.

In addition to platelet basic protein (a precursor of platelet factor 4 and β-thromboglobulin) and neutrophil activating peptide 2 (NAP-2), connective tissue activating peptide-III (CTAP-III), a platelet granule peptide with potent activities related to fibroblast growth, wound repair, inflammation and neoplasia, is derived by proteolytic processing from its CXC chemokine precursor, leukocyte-derived growth factor.[1,2] CTAP-III and NAP-2 are heparanases whose growth promoting activities could result from solubilization of heparan sulfate and any bound growth factors in the extracellular matrix.[3] In addition to other chemokines, CTAP-III is one of the family of molecules formerly referred to as "histamine release factors."[4] In the late-phase reaction characteristic of allergic states, CTAP-III (as well as the other chemokines) can stimulate or inhibit histamine release; whether these chemokines are agonistic or antagonistic is perhaps dependent on their relative concentrations, the temporal pattern of release and the degree of responsiveness of localized basophils and mast cells.[4] The neutrophil activating potential of CTAP-III provides a key link between platelet activation and neutrophil recruitment and stimulation, which is a key feature of inflammatory reactions in allergic states. See in this Chapter: **Histamine Release Factors**, **Histamine Release Inhibitory Factors**, **Neutrophil Activating Peptide 2**, **Platelet Factor-4** and Chapter 6: **Chemokines**.

REFERENCES
1. Iida N, Haisa M, Igarashi A, Pencev D, Grotendorst GR. Leukocyte-derived growth factor links the PDGF and CXC chemokine families of peptides. FASEB J 1996;10:1336-45.
2. Power CA, Clemetson JM, Clemetson KJ, Wells TNC. Chemokine and chemokine receptor mRNA expression in human platelets. Cytokine 1995;7:479-82.
3. Hoogewerf AJ, Leone JW, Reardon IM, et al. CXC chemokines connective tissue activating peptide-III and neutrophil activating peptide-2 are heparin/heparan sulfate-degrading enzymes. J Biol Chem 1995;270:3268-77.
4. Kuna P, Reddigari SR, Rucinski D, Schall TJ, Kaplan AP. Chemokines of the α, β-subclass inhibit human basophil's responsiveness to monocyte chemotactic and activating factor/monocyte chemoattractant protein-1. J Allergy Clin Immunol 1995;95:574-86.

Defensins

Guo Qiu Shen, M.D.

Defensins (human neutrophil proteins 1-4) are amphipathic, carbohydrate-free, cytotoxic membrane-active antimicrobial molecules. Three of the defensin peptides (HP-1, HP-2, and HP-3) are almost identical in sequence. HP-1 and HP-3 are 30 amino acids long and differ only at the first amino acid, which is Ala in HP-1 and Asp in HP-3. In contrast, sequences of HP-4, P-5, and HP-6 are very different, sharing only 10 amino acids with other HP peptides.[1] HP-1 and HP-2 are chemotactic for monocytes; whereas, HP-3 is not.[2-6] The high concentrations of HP-1 - 4 (25–200 µg/mL) exhibit antimicrobial and/or viricidal properties *in vitro;* HP-4 showing the greatest defensin activity and HP-3 the least.[7,8] The low concentrations of mixed HP-1, 2, and 3 (1–25 µg/mL) affect mammalian cell growth; they are cytotoxic for some cell lines but promote the growth of others. The functions of HP-5 and HP-6 are unknown.[9,10]

Serum antibodies from patients with onchocerciasis were reacted to a 2.5 kd antigen present in extracts of *Onchocerca volvulus*. The amino acid sequence suggested identity of this antigen with human defensins. The study suggests a link between formation of autoantibodies to defensin and enhanced immune reactivity towards the parasite.[11]

REFERENCES
1. Lehrer RI, Ganz T, Selsted ME. Defensins: endogenous antibiotic peptides of animal cells [Review]. Cell 1991;64:229-30.

2. Boman HG. Antibacterial peptides: key components needed in immunity [Review]. Cell 1991;65:205-7.
3. Spitznagel JK. Antibiotic proteins of human neutrophils [Review]. J Clin Invest 1990;86:1381-6.
4. Lichtenstein A. Mechanism of mammalian cell lysis mediated by peptide defensins. Evidence for an initial alteration of the plasma membrane. J Clin Invest 1991;88:93-100.
5. Mars WM, Patmasiriwat P, Maity T, Huff V, Weil MM, Saunders GF. Inheritance of unequal numbers of the genes encoding the human neutrophil defensins HP-1 and HP-3. J Biol Chem 1995;270:30371-6.
6. Zhu QZ, Singh AV, Bateman A, Esch F, Solomon S. The corticostatic (anti-ACTH) and cytotoxic activity of peptides isolated from fetal, adult and tumor-bearing lung. J Steroid Biochem 1987;27:1017-22.
7. Wilde CG, Griffith JE, Marra MN, Snable JL, Scott RW. Purification and characterization of human neutrophil peptide 4, a novel member of the defensin family. J Biol Chem 1989;264:11200-3.
8. Lehrer RI, Ganz T, Szklarek D, Selsted ME. Modulation of the in vitro candidacidal activity of human neutrophil defensins by target cell metabolism and divalent cations. J Clin Invest 1988;81:1829-35.
9. Singh A, Bateman A, Zhu QZ, Shimasaki S, Esch F, Solomon S. Structure of a novel human granulocyte peptide with anti-ACTH activity. Biochem Biophys Res Commun 1988;155:524-9.
10. Okrent DG, Lichtenstein AK, Ganz T. Direct cytotoxicity of polymorphonuclear leukocyte granule proteins to human lung-derived cells and endothelial cells. Am Rev Respir Dis 1990;141:179-85.
11. Gallin MY, Jacobi AB, Büttner DW, Schönberger Ö, Marti T, Erttmann KD. Human autoantibody to defensin: disease association with hyperreactive onchocerciasis (Sowda). J Exp Med 1995;182:41-7.

Eosinophil Cationic Protein

Emmanuel A. Ojo-Amaize, Ph.D.

Eosinophil cationic protein (ECP), a highly basic, single chain, zinc-containing protein present in the granules of eosinophils,[1] has cytotoxic, helminthotoxic, ribonuclease and bactericidal activities. The four principal eosinophil granule proteins include ECP, major basic protein (MBP), eosinophil-derived neurotoxin (EDN) and eosinophil peroxidase (EPO).[2] Upon activation of heart mast cells, ECP and MBP stimulate the release of preformed histamine and the *de novo* synthesis of vasoactive and proinflammatory mediators (PGD2) from human heart tissue.[2] ECP is elevated in acute graft rejection[3] and atopic dermatitis;[4] whereas, serum MBP concentrations are increased in the sera of patients with systemic sclerosis.[5] In addition to its involvement in several disease states, MBP can act as a cytostimulant and as a toxin;[6] whereas, ECP, EPO, EDN and MBP possess a wide range of biologic activities, including the ability to activate other cells such as basophils, neutrophils and platelets.[7]

A sensitive EIA is available for ECP detection in serum, urine and CSF.[1] A flow cytometric method can detect intracellular eosinophil proteins in peripheral blood and bone marrow eosinophils.[8] See in this Chapter: **Eosinophil Granule Major Basic Protein.**

REFERENCES
1. Reimert CM, Venge P, Kharazmi A, Bendtzen K. Detection of eosinophil cationic protein (ECP) by an enzyme-linked immunosorbent assay. J Immunol Method 1991;138:285-90.
2. Patella V, de Crescenzo G, Marino I, et al. Eosinophil granule proteins activate human heart mast cells. J Immunol 1996;157:1219-25.
3. Riise GC, Schersten H, Nilsson F, Ryd W, Andersson BA. Activation of eosinophils and fibroblasts assessed by eosinophil cationic protein and hyaluronan in BAL. Association with acute rejection in lung transplant recipients. Chest 1996;110:89-96.
4. Wakita H, Sakamoto T, Tokura Y, Takigawa M. E-selectin and vascular cell adhesion molecule-1 as critical adhesion molecules for infiltration of T lymphocytes and eosinophils in atomic dermatitis. J Cutan Pathol 1994;21:33-9.
5. Cox D, Earle L, Jimenez SA, et al. Elevated levels of eosinophil major basic protein in the sera of patients with systemic sclerosis. Arthritis Rheum 1995;38:939-45.
6. Popken-Harris P, Thomas L, Oxvig C, et al. Biochemical properties, activities, and presence of biologic fluids of eosinophil granule major basic protein. J Allergy Clin Immunol 1994;94(6 Pt 2):1282-9.
7. Kita H, Abu-Ghazaleh RI, Sur S, Gleich GJ. Eosinophil major basic protein induces degranulation and IL-8 production by human eosinophils. J Immunol 1995;154:4749-58.
8. Krug N, Thurau AM, Lackie P, et al. A flow cytometric method for the detection of intracellular basic proteins in unseparated peripheral blood and bone marrow eosinophils. J Immunol Methods 1996;190:245-54.

Eosinophil Granule Major Basic Protein

Emmanuel A. Ojo-Amaize, Ph.D.

Eosinophil granule major basic protein (EGMBP), an arginine-rich polypeptide released from the granules of eosinophils,[1] is a potent toxin for helminths and some mammalian cells. EGMBP plays an important role in late-phase reactions in allergy and asthma,[2] and in late-phase cutaneous reactions to allergens such as dust mites.[3] EGMBP might be important in endomyocardial damage[4] caused by the cardiac localization of eosinophil granule proteins.[4] Eosinophilopoietic cytokines, such as IL-3, GM-CSF and IL-5, activate eosinophils and prolong their survival.[5] These cytokines are present in the airways of patients with bronchial asthma[5] and contribute to eosinophil activation, which in turn, results in epithelial damage.[5] Inhibition of EGMBP release by IFN-α could be the basis for the beneficial effects of IFN-α in patients with hypereosinophilic syndromes.[6] EGMBP from infiltrating eosinophils (in skin lesions of atopic dermatitis) is usually measured by immunohistochemical analysis.[7] See in this Chapter: **Eosinophil Cationic Protein.**

REFERENCES
1. Barker RL, Gundel RH, Gleich GJ, et al. Acidic polyamino acids inhibit human eosinophil granule major basic protein toxicity. Evidence for a functional role for ProMBP. J Clin Invest 1991;88:798-805.
2. Oh NL, Gleich GJ, Peterson EA, et al. Assessment of eosinophil and neutrophil participation in atopic dermatitis: comparison with the IgE-mediated late-phase reaction. J Allergy Clin Immunol 1994;94:120-8.
3. Wakugawa M, Nakagawa H, Yamada N, Tamaki K. Chronologic analysis of eosinophil granule protein deposition and cell adhesion molecule expression in mite allergen-induced dermatitis in atopic subjects. Int Arch Allergy Immunol 1996;111(Suppl 1):5-11.
4. Patella V, de Crescenzo G, Marino I, et al. Eosinophil granule proteins activate human heart mast cells. J Immunol 1996;157:1219-25.
5. Adachi T, Motojima S, Hirata A, et al. Eosinophil apoptosis caused by theophylline, glucocorticoids, and macrolides after stimulation with IL-5. J Allergy Clin Immunol 1996;98:S308-S215.
6. Aldebert D, Lamkhioued B, DeSaint C, et al. Eosinophils express a functional receptor for interferon alpha: inhibitory role of interferon alpha on the release of mediators. Blood 1996;87:2354-60.
7. Wakita H, Sakamoto T, Tokura Y, Takigawa M. E-selecting and vascular cell adhesion molecule-1 as critical adhesion molecules for infiltration of T lymphocytes and eosinophils in atopic dermatitis. J Cutan Pathol 1994;21:33-9.

Eosinophil and Neutrophil Chemotactic Activities

Emmanuel A. Ojo-Amaize, Ph.D.

Factors with chemotactic activities for eosinophils and neutrophils (ECA, NCA) are found in bronchoalveolar lavage fluid (BALF) of some asthmatic patients.[1] ECA is important in initiating early atopic dermatitis lesions, and is induced by transepidermal mite allergen permeation.[2] In addition to their involvement in atopic disorders, eosinophils are associated with acute rejection in kidney and liver grafts, as assessed by eosinophil cationic protein.[3] Eosinophil major basic protein interacts with IL-1 and transforming growth factor-β to upregulate lung fibroblasts to produce IL-6-type cytokine production.[4] Upon stimulation with C5a, eosinophils produce significant amounts of H_2O_2 as measured by chemiluninescence (CL).[5] Thus, C5a, generated after activation of the complement system, could be of major importance for the eosinophil activation observed in eisonophil-related diseases.[5] Eosinophil activation can also be detected by flow cytometric methods.[6]

Increased susceptibility to bacterial infection in neonates can be due to defective adherence and migration of neonatal neutrophils.[7] Neutrophil-activating peptide ENA-78, a novel chemotactic cytokine and a member of the chemokine family of proinflammatory polypeptides, shares sequence similarity with IL-8 and GRO-α.[8] ENA-78 is a potent upregulator of Mac-1 cell surface expression[8] and is detected in cystic fibrosis lung.[8] ENA-78 mRNA levels are increased in human pulmonary inflammation.[8]

Laboratory methods used for the assessment of neutrophil activation include CL,[5] flow cytometry[6] and nitroblue tetrazolium reduction test.[9]

REFERENCES
1. Sato E, Koyama S, Nomura H, Kubo K, Sekiguchi M. Bradykinin stimulates alveolar macrophages to release neutrophil, monocyte, and eosinophil chemotactic activity. J Immunol 1996;157:3122-9.
2. Wakugawa M, Nakagawa H, Yamada N, Tamaki K. Chronologic analysis of eosinophil granule protein deposition and cell adhesion molecule expression in mite allergen-induced dermatitis in atopic subjects. Int Arch Allergy Immunol 1996;111(Suppl 1):5-11.
3. Riise GC, Schersten H, Nilsson F, Ryd W, Andersson BA. Activation of eosinophils and fibroblasts assessed by eosinophil cationic protein and hyaluronan in BAL. Association with acute rejection in lung transplant recipients. Chest 1996;110:89-96.
4. Rochester CL, Ackerman SJ, Zheng T, Elias JA. Eosinophil-fibroblast interactions. Granule major basic protein interacts with IL-1 and transforming growth factor-β in the stimulation of lung fibroblast IL-6-type cytokine production. J Immunol 1996;156:4449-56.
5. Zeck-Kapp G, Kroegel C, Riede UN, Kapp A. Mechanisms of human eosinophil activation by complement protein C5a and platelet-activating factor: similar functional responses are accompanied by different morphologic alterations. Allergy 1995;50:34-47.
6. Krug N, Thurau AM, Lackie P, et al. A flow cytometric method for the detection of intracellular basic proteins in unseparated peripheral blood and bone marrow eosinophils. J Immunol Method 1996;190:245-54.
7. Kjeldsen L, Sengelor H, Lollike K, Borregaard N. Granules and secretory vesicles in human neonatal netrophils. Pediatr Res 1996;40:120-9.
8. Bozic CR, Gerard NP, Gerard C. Receptor binding specificity and pulmonary gene expression of the neutrophil-activating peptide ENA-78. Am J Respir Cell Mol Biol 1996;14:302-8.
9. Perlingeiro RC, Queiroz ML. Measurement of the respiratory burst and chemotaxis in polymorphonuclear leukocytes from mercury-exposed workers. Hum Exp Toxicol 1995;14:281-6.

Histamine Release Assays

Douglas C. Aziz, M.D., Ph.D.

Mononuclear cell preparations of peripheral blood are targets for histamine release assays (HRA). Histamine production by basophils can be measured under unstimulated conditions or after stimulation by cytokines and/or anti-IgE, C5a, and histamine release factors.[1] Several cytokines (IL-3, IL-5, GM-CSF, CTAP-III and NAP-2) can prime basophils to release histamine so that the response to anti-IgE is enhanced. In a subset of patients, representing 4-13% of the allergic population, the IgE-mediated release of histamine from basophils is dependent on, rather than merely enhanced by, these cytokines.[2] These anti-IgE-non-releasers will respond to agents such as f-Met-Leu-Pro (FMLP), which bypasses the IgE receptor pathway. Serum IgE concentrations and basophil receptor occupancy are not involved in the mechanism of histamine release by basophils, but dependent on cell-imminent mechanisms in basophils, which can be altered in selective atopic patients.[3] This could explain why HRA are most useful in situations in which skin testing and RAST perform suboptimally, particularly in patients with urticaria and atopic dermatitis where the correlation between disease and IgE concentration is weak. Studies with mite allergen suggest that an intrinsic cellular property and IgE antibody concentrations on the basophil surface determine histamine release.[4] A cutaneous microdialysis method is used to measure substance-P-induced histamine release.[5] This microdialysis method should prove to be a valuable assessment of histamine release and other biochemical events *in vivo* in intact human skin together with clinical observations (i.e., wheal, flare, and itch responses). HRA are most useful in patients with urticaria, asthma and atopic dermatitis.

REFERENCES
1. Grant JA, Alam R, Lett-Brown MA. Histamine-releasing factors and inhibitors: historical perspectives and possible implications in human illness. J Allergy Clin Immunol 1991;88:683-93.
2. Black KM, Lussier AM, Gion WR, Kasaian MT. Cytokine priming of human basophils: description of allergen "nonreleasers". Int Arch Allergy Immunol 1996;111:142-51.
3. Bischoff SC, Zwahlen R, Stucki M, et al. Basophil histamine release and leukotriene production in response to anti-IgE and anti-IgE receptor antibodies. Int Arch Allergy Immunol 1996;110:261-71.

4. Mita H, Yasueda H, Ishii T, Akiyama K. IgE-mediated basophil releasability is influenced by intrinsic factors and by IgE on the cell surface. Allergy 1995;50:952-8.
5. Petersen LJ, Poulsen LK, Sondergaard J, Skov PS. The use of cutaneous microdialysis to measure substance P-induced histamine release in intact human skin in vivo. J Allergy Clin Immunol 1994;94:773-83.

Histamine Release Factors

Douglas C. Aziz, M.D., Ph.D.

Histamine release factors (HRF) comprise a group of protein cytokines which cause release of histamine from basophils and mast cells.[1] The 12 kd HRF resembles connective tissue activating peptide-III (CTAP-III) and its degradation product, which is termed neutrophil activating peptide 2 (NAP-2).[1] Sera from 27% of patients with chronic idiopathic urticaria (CIU) contain a factor with histamine-releasing activity in the IgG fraction which should prove to be a useful marker in positive CIU patients because its presence correlates well with disease activity.[2,3] See in this Chapter: **Connective Tissue Activating Peptide-III** and **Neutrophil Activating Peptide 2**.

REFERENCES
1. Grant JA, Alam R, Lett-Brown MA. Histamine-releasing factors and inhibitors: historical perspectives and possible implications in human illness. J Allergy Clin Immunol 1991;88:683-93.
2. Tanus T, Atkins PC, Zweiman B. Comparison of serum histamine-releasing activity and clinical manifestations in chronic idiopathic urticaria. Clin Diagn Lab Immunol 1996;3:135-7.
3. Zweiman B, Valenzano M, Atkins PC, Tanus T, Getsy JA. Characteristics of histamine-releasing activity in the sera of patients with chronic idiopathic urticaria. J Allergy Clin Immunol 1996;98:89-8.

Histamine Release Inhibitory Factor: See Chapter 6: Chemokines.

Intercellular Adhesion Molecule-1 (CD54)

Alaa E. Ahmed, Ph.D.

Intercellular adhesion molecule-1 (ICAM-1), a member of the immunoglobulin gene superfamily of cell adhesion molecules, is expressed by several cell types including leukocytes and endothelial cells.[1] ICAM-1 can be upregulated in a cell-specific manner by several cytokines such as TNF-α, IL-1, and INF-γ. The upregulation is inhibited by glucocorticoids.[1,2] ICAM-1 ligands include the membrane-bound integrin receptors LFA-1 and Mac-1 on leukocytes, CD43, fibrinogen, the matrix factor hyaluronan, rhinoviruses and *Plasmodium falciparum* malaria-infected erythrocytes.[1,3]

ICAM-1 plays a major role in the inflammatory response and in T-cell mediated host responses by acting as a costimulatory molecule on antigen-presenting cells to activate MHC class II restricted T cells and on other cell types in association with MHC class I to activate cytotoxic T cells.[4] On endothelial cells it has an important role in the migration of activated leukocytes to the site of injury.[5] The clinical significance of soluble forms of ICAM-1 (sICAM-1) found in serum in many pathological conditions, as yet, is unclear.[1] Exhaustion of ICAM-1 expression could be a contributing factor to the clinical manifestations of such diverse disorders as malignancies (lymphomas), inflammation (asthma), atherosclerosis and neurological disease.[1]

ICAM-1 is the cellular receptor for a subgroup of rhinoviruses;[1] a soluble form of ICAM-1 inhibits infection of cells by the rhinoviruses[1] which cause 50% of common colds.

REFERENCES
1. van de Stolpe A, van der Saag PT. Intercellular adhesion molecule-1. J Mol Med 1996;74:13-33.
2. Tosi MF, Stark JM, Smith CW, et al. Induction of ICAM-1 expression on human airway epithelial cells by inflammatory cytokines: effects on neutrophil-epithelial cell adhesion. Am J Respir Cell Mol Biol 1992;7:214-21.

3. De Fougerolles AR, Qin X, Springer TA. Characterization of the function of intercellular adhesion molecule (ICAM)-3 and comparison with ICAM-1 and ICAM-2 in immune responses. J Exp Med 1995;179:619-29.
4. Ybarrondo B, O'Rourke AM, Brian AA, et al. Contribution of lymphocyte function-associated-1/intracellular adhesion molecule-1 binding to the adhesion/signalling cascade of cytotoxic T lymphocyte activation. J Exp Med 1994;179:359-63.
5. Muller WA, Weigel SA, Deng X, et al. PECAM-1 is required for tensendothelial migration of leukocytes. J Exp Med 1993;178:449-60.

Leukocyte Adhesion Molecules

Alaa E. Ahmed, Ph.D.

Leukocyte adhesion is an essential function for vascular endothelium aggregation, chemotaxis, cytotoxicity, binding of iC3b-coated particles, lymphocyte proliferation and phagocytosis.[1] Leukocyte cell adhesion molecules (Leu-CAMs) belong to three main families: the selectins, integrins, and immunoglobulin superfamily (Table).[2] Soluble forms of Leu-CAM are reported to be elevated in a variety of autoimmune disorders; however, their clinical utility is unclear.

The Selectin Family				
Molecule	**Size**	**Expression**	**Ligand**	**Role**
L-selectin	74 kd	Leukocytes	CD34 CD54	Lymphocyte Binding, Leukocyte Rolling
P-selectin	140 kd	Endothelium Platelets	SLe^{x,a} PSGL-1 ?L-selectin	PMN,Mon Recruitment
E-selectin	115 kd	Activated endothelium	SLe^{x,a} PSGL-1	PMN,Mon Recruitment

The Integrin Family			
Molecule	**Size**	**Expression**	**Ligand**
α4β1 (VLA-4)	150/130	B, T cells	VCAM-1 Fibronectin
α4β7 (LPAM-1)	150/120	B, T cells	VCAM-1 MAdCAM-1
αLβ2 (LFA-1)	80/95	B, T cells PMN,Mono	ICAM-1, -2, -3
αMβ2 (Mac-1, CR3)	165/95	Mono,PMN	ICAM-1 iC3b, FX Fibrinogen
αXβ2 (P150/95)	150/95	Mono,PMN	iC3b, Fibrinogen

The Immunoglobulin Superfamily				
Molecule	**Size**	**Expression**	**Ligand**	**Role**
ICAM-1 (CD54)	90–115 kd	varies	FLA-1 αLβ2	Adhesion Activation Arrest Transmigration
ICAM-2 (CD102)	55/65	Endothelium Lymphocytes	LFA-1 αLβ2	Adhesion Activation Arrest
VCAM-1 (CD106)	110 kd	Endothelium Macrophages Others	VLA-4 α4β1 LPAM-1 α4β7	Adhesion Activation Arrest

The Immunoglobulin Superfamily				
Molecule	Size	Expression	Ligand	Role
ICAM-3	58/66	Endothelium	LPAM-1 L-selectin	Adhesion Activation Arrest
PECAM-1 (CD31)	120/130	Endothelium Platelets Lymphocytes	PECAM-1	Transmigration

Leu-CAM deficiencies, also known as leukocyte adhesion deficiencies, are partial or complete inherited deficiencies of cell surface expression of CD18 and CD11a-c. These deficiencies prevent granulocytes from reaching extravascular sites of inflammation. Patients consequently experience recurrent infections and even death in severe cases (usually before the age of 2).[3,4]

REFERENCES
1. Hogg N, Berlin C. Structure and function of adhesion receptors in leukocytes trafficking. Immunol Today 1995;16:327-30.
2. Tedder TF, Steeber DA, Chen A, Engel P. The selectins: vascular adhesion molecules. FASEB J 1995;9:866-73.
3. Bazil V. Physiological enzymatic cleavage of leukocyte membrane molecules. Immunol Today 1995;16:135-40.
4. Arnaout MA, Dana N, Gupta SK, Tenen DG, Fathallah DM. Point mutations impairing cell surface expression of the common β subunit (CD18) in a patient with leukocyte adhesion molecule (Leu-CAM) deficiency. J Clin Invest 1990;85:977-81.

Lymphocyte Antigen Stimulation Test

Emmanuel A. Ojo-Amaize, Ph.D.

Lymphocyte antigen stimulation assays for *in vitro* assessment of impaired cellular immunity are useful in evaluating patients with genetic or acquired immunodeficiencies, bacterial and viral infections, cancer, several autoimmune disorders, transplantation-related disorders,[1]antisperm antibodies[4] and individuals with previous exposure to a variety of antigens,[3] allergens,[4] pathogens[5] and metals/chemicals.[6-9] Defects in the ability of lymphocytes to respond to antigenic stimulation are reported in AIDS,[10] malaria[11] and patients with stage III giant cell tumors.[3] Lymphocyte antigen stimulation is routinely measured by [^{3}H]-thymidine uptake. However, comparison of a flow cytometric assay (based on expression of the activation antigen CD69) with [^{3}H]-thymidine incorporation reveals that both assays detect lymphocyte responses to antigenic stimuli.[10] Supernatants from antigen-stimulated cultures can be assessed for cytokine production by EIA.

Lymphocyte antigen stimulation assays are valuable tools for the determination of hypersensitivity reactions to beryllium,[7] silicates, silica and silicone,[6] mercury[12] and for monitoring cytokine shifts (T_H1-T_H2) following immunotherapy.[6] See in this Chapter: **Lymphocyte Mitogen Stimulation Test.**

REFERENCES
1. Abbas AB, Lichtman AH, Pober JS, editors. Cellular and Molecular Immunology. 3rd edition. Philadelphia: W.B. Saunders Company, 1997.
2. Naz RK, Chaudhry A, Witkin SS. Lymphocyte proliferative response to fertilization antigen in patients with antisperm antibodies. Am J Obstet Gynecol 1990;163:610-3.
3. Muscolo DL, Ayerza MA. Lymphocyte *in vitro* response to human giant cell tumors. Clin Orthop 1996;326:55-62.
4. McHugh SM, Deighton J, Stewart AG, et al. Bee venom immunotherapy induces a shift in cytokine responses from a TH-2 to a TH-1 dominant pattern: comparison of rush and conventional immunotherapy. Clin Exp Allergy 1995;25:828-38.

5. Neustock P, Kruse A, Bein G, et al. Failure to detect type I interferon production in human umbilical cord vein endothelial cells after viral exposure. J Interferon Cytokine Res 1995;15:129-35.

6. Ojo-Amaize EA, Conte V, Lin H-C, et al. Silicone-specific blood lymphocyte response in women with silicone breast implants. Clin Diagn Lab Immunol 1994;1:689-95.

7. Ojo-Amaize EA, Agopian MS, Peter JB. Novel in vitro method for identification of individuals at risk for beryllium hypersensitivity. Clin Diagn Lab Imunol 1994;1:164-71.

8. Kapsenberg MD, Wierenga EA, Stiedema EM, Bos JD. TH1 lymphokine production profiles of nickel-specific CD4$^+$ T-lymphocyte clones from nickel contact allergic and non-allergic individuals. J Invest Dermatol 1992;98:59-63.

9. Romagnoli P, Spinas GA, Sinigaglia F. Gold-specific T-cells in rheumatoid arthritis patients treated with gold. J Clin Invest 1992;89:254-8.

10. Krowka JF, Cuevas B, Maron DC, et al. Expression of CD69 after in vitro stimulation: a rapid method for quantitating impaired lymphocyte responses in HIV-infected individuals. J Acquir Immune Defic Syndr Hum Retrovirol 1995;11:95-104.

11. Riley EM, Jobe O, Blackman M, et al. Plasmodium falciparum schizont sonic extracts suppress lymphoproliferative responses to mitogens and antigens in malaria-immune adults. Infect Immun 1989;57:3181-8.

12. Coers W, Vos TWM, Van Der Meide PH, et al. Interferon-gamma (IFN-γ) and IL-4 expressed during mercury-induced membranous nephropathy are toxic for cultured podocytes. Clin Exp Immunol 1995;102:297-307.

Lymphocyte Mitogen Stimulation Test

Emmanuel A. Ojo-Amaize, Ph.D.

Lymphocyte mitogen stimulation assays are used for *in vitro* assessment of cellular immunity in patients with immunodeficiency,[1] autoimmunity,[2] infectious diseases,[3] cancer[4] and chemical-induced hypersensitivity reactions.[5] Lymphocytes from healthy human subjects have receptors for mitogens such as the plant lectin concanavalin A (Con A), pokeweed mitogen (PWM), the protein A component of *Staphylococcus aureus* Cowan strain I (SpA) and chemicals.[5-7] Lymphocytes respond to these mitogens (substances that stimulate large numbers of lymphocytes without prior sensitization and in contrast to antigens do not require a sensitized host). Both B cells and T cells can be stimulated with mitogens.[6] Inability of lymphocytes to respond to mitogens is a sign of impaired cell-mediated or humoral immunity.[1,8]

There is a good correlation between CD4$^+$ T-cell subset numbers and mitogenic response to PWM at different disease states in patients with HIV infection.[8]

[³H]-thymidine uptake is the gold standard for measuring lymphocyte mitogen stimulation.[6] However, a newer and more practical method utilizing supravital stains[9] shows a good correlation with [³H]-thymidine uptake. Flow cytometry was also recently applied to analyze proliferation of cultured cells in response to stimulation with mitogen.[10] See in this Chapter: **Lymphocyte Antigen Stimulation Test.**

REFERENCES

1. Edelman AS, Zolla-Pazner S. Response of mononuclear cells from HIV-infected patients to B-cell mitogens: correlation with immunological and clinical features of disease progression. AIDS 1990;4:859-64.

2. Kalman B, Olsson O, Link H, Kam-Hansen S. Estradiol potentiates pokeweed mitogen-induced B cell stimulation in multiple sclerosis and healthy subjects. Acta Neurol Scand 1989;79:340-6.

3. Ponniah S, Abraham SN, Dockter ME, Wall CD, Endres RO. Mitogenic stimulation of human B lymphocytes by the mannose-specific adhesion on Escherichia coli type I fimbriae. J Immunol 1989;142:992-8.

4. Paletta E, Stockert RJ, McManus M, et al. Hodgkin's cell lectin, a lymphocyte adhesion molecule and mitogen. J Immunol 1989;143:2850-7.

5. Ueki A, Yamaguchi M, Ueki H, et al. Polyclonal human T-cell activation by silicate in vitro. Immunology 1994;82:332-5.

6. Abbas AK, Lichtman AH, Pober JS, editors. Cellular and Molecular Immunology. 3rd Edition. Philadelphia: W.B. Saunders Company, 1997.

7. Malave I, Rodriguez J, Araujo Z, Rojas I. Effect of zinc on the proliferative response of human lymphocytes: mechanism of its mitogenic action. Immunopharmacology 1990;20:1-10.
8. Bansal AS, Moran A, Potter M, Taylor R, Haeney MR, Mandal BK. Lymphocyte transformation responses to phytohaemagglutinin and pokeweed mitogen in patients at different stages of HIV infection: are they worth measuring? J Clin Pathol 1993;46:846-8.
9. Giorgio A, Rambaldi M, Iaquinto G, et al. A simple and rapid method to evaluate lymphocyte response to mitogens. Microbiologica 1989;12:151-5.
10. Yamamura Y, Rodriguez N, Schwartz A, Eylar E, Yano N. Anti-CD4 cytotoxic T ymphocyte (CTL) activity in HIV+ patients: flow cytometric analysis. Cell Mol Biol 1995;41(Suppl 1):S133-44.

Lymphocyte Toxicity Assay

Emmanuel A. Ojo-Amaize, Ph.D.

Lymphocyte toxicity assay (LTA), a promising test for assessing adverse reactions to drugs, particularly anticonvulsants, is entirely distinct from the cytotoxicity or cell killing/tumoricidal assays utilized in the assessment of NK or CD8[+] cytotoxic suppressor cell function, respectively.[1] In LTA, incubation with hepatic microsomes is thought to metabolize the drug to the *in vivo* metabolite which in turn kills lymphocytes from sensitized patients but not from controls. Lymphocytes derived from non-reactive individuals do not show significant lymphocyte toxicity. LTA is of added value over the lymphocyte proliferation assays only in a select patient group and is of little value in cases where skin or RAST testing can be carried out.[2]

Certain human lymphocyte enzymes, such as neuropathy target esterase (NTE), are promising markers in clinical toxicology.[3] Thus, LTA is gradually being replaced by such enzyme assays which employ lymphocyte esterases and hydroxylases for evaluation of toxic neuropathies.[3] Another test, sister chromatid exchange, can be very useful in the assessment of antimutagenic activity of certain agents cultured with human blood-derived lymphocytes.[4]

Because toxic insult is no longer assumed to be the direct cause of death, it is now thought that molecular damage can be a start signal in a pathway that converges on a limited number of ubiquitous cellular transformations that precedes cell death.[5] The cascade of cellular events that leads to cell death is believed to be programmed. This programmed cell death, known as apoptosis, is thought to be standardized from cell to cell, regardless of the manner by which it is induced.[6] Apoptosis is measured by DNA fragmentation analysis, flow cytometry,[7] and by the use of antinuclear matrix antibodies.[8]

REFERENCES
1. Jiang X, Khursigara G, Rubin RL. Transformation of lupus-inducing drugs to cytotoxic products by activated neutrophils. Science 1994;266:810-3.
2. Shear NH, Spieberg SP. Anticonvulsant hypersensitivity syndrome: *In vitro* assessment of risk. J Clin Invest 1988;82:1826-32.
3. Fournier L, Musard D, Lecorsier A. Lymphocyte esterases and hydroxylases in neurotoxicology. Vet Hum Toxicol 1996;38:190-5.
4. Gasiorowski K, Szyba K, Brokos B, Kozubek A. Antimutagenic activity of alkyresorcinols from cereal grains. Cancer Lett 1996;106:109-15.
5. Tomei LD, Cope FO. Introduction, apoptosis: the molecular basis of cell death. In: Tomei LD, Cope FO, editors. Current communications in cell and molecular biology. Volume 3. New York: Cold Spring Harbor Laboratory Press, 1991:1-4.
6. Strand S, Hofmann WJ, Hug H, et al. Lymphocyte apoptosis induced by CD95 (APO-1/Fas) ligand-expressing tumor cells - a mechanism of immune evasion? Nature Medicine 1996;2:1361-6.
7. Aten J, Prigent P, Poncet P, et al. Mercuric chloride-induced programmed cell death of a murine T cell hybridoma. I. Effect of the proto-oncogene *bcl*-2. Cell Immunol 1995;161:98-106.
8. Miller T, Beausang LA, Meneghini M, Lidgard G. Death-induced changes to the nuclear matrix: the use of antinuclear matrix antibodies to study agents of apoptosis. Biotechniques 1993;15:1042-7.

Mast Cell Tryptase

Douglas C. Aziz, M.D., Ph.D.

Mast cell tryptase, a serine protease found in the secretory granules of mast cells and released along with histamine during mast cell activation, has several biologic activities relevant to allergy and asthma including: prevention of coagulation at sites of immediate hypersensitivity reactions by inactivation of fibrinogen and by complex formation with heparin; activation of latent collagenase via the activation of another matrix metalloproteinase-3; augmentation of smooth muscle contractile responses to histamine; generation of C3a; and stimulation of secretory activity in the airways. Serum tryptase is a clinical indicator of diseases of mast-cell activation such as systemic anaphylaxis or mastocytosis, and probably a better *in vitro* marker of anaphylaxis than histamine because tryptase has a slower release and is more stable. Timing of blood drawing for histamine and tryptase is critical for the postmortem diagnosis of acute anaphylaxis.[6] Unlike histamine, which demonstrates a rapid rise-peaking at about 5 minutes post anaphylaxis, and returning to baseline within 15 to 60 minutes-tryptase concentrations increase later, peak at 1 to 2 hrs and remain elevated for several hours. The half-life of tryptase is 90 minutes, and it takes at least 15 minutes to have detectable concentrations.[1] The best time to measure tryptase is 1 to 2 hrs but not >6 after the reaction.[1] In patients with severe anaphylaxis after bee sting challenge, maximal serum tryptase is 406 ± 1062 U/L (range = 1.8 to 4400 U/L).[2] Subjects with no reaction and unexposed to the bee sting all have serum tryptase concentrations below 1 U/L.[2] In anaphylaxis, both α- and β-tryptase are elevated; in systemic mastocytosis, only the α-form is elevated.[3]

Most studies indicate that tryptase is elevated in postmortem blood after severe anaphylaxis, and is a reliable postmortem indicator of fatal anaphylaxis. Tryptase concentrations are elevated above 10 µg/mL in up to 13% of unexplained deaths.[4] Witnessed deaths due to anaphylaxis are associated with elevated (>12 ng/mL) concentrations in 100% of hymenoptera sting fatalities, 100% of therapeutic agent anaphylaxis, and 75% of deaths due to food allergy.[5] Mild or moderate anaphylaxis, and samples drawn at the inappropriate time postanaphylaxis, can be negative. Conversely, elevated postmortem tryptase occurs in the absence of anaphylaxis and therefore should not be used as the sole criterion for the postmortem diagnosis of anaphylaxis.[6] Other important clinical factors are the atopic disposition of the deceased, the temporal relationship between exposure to the allergen and death, and the finding of allergen-specific IgE.[7] Postmortem allergen-specific-IgE concentrations should also be obtained if possible.

REFERENCES

1. Laroche D, Vergnaud M-C, Sillard B, Soufarapis H, Bricard H. Biochemical markers of anaphylactoid reactions to drugs. Anesthesiology 1991;75:945-9.
2. van der Linden P-W G, Hack CE, Poortman J, Vivié-KippYC, Struyvenberg A, van der Zwan JK. Insect-sting challenge in 138 patients: relation between clinical severity of anaphylaxis and mast cell activation. J Allergy Clin Immunol 1992;90:110-8.
3. Schwartz LB, Sakai K, Bradford TR, et al. The α form of human tryptase is the predominant type present in blood at baseline in normal subjects and is elevated in those with systemic mastocytosis. J Clin Invest 1995;96:2702-10.
4. Schwartz HJ, Yuninger JW, Schwartz LB. Is unrecognized anaphylaxis a cause of sudden unexpected death? Clin Exp Allergy 1995;25:866-70.
5. Yuninger JW, Nelson DR, Squillace DL, et al. Laboratory investigation of deaths due to anaphylaxis. J Forensic Sci 1991;36:857-65.
6. Randall B, Butts J, Halsey JF. Elevated postmortem tryptase in the absence of anaphylaxis. J Forensic Sci 1995;40:208-11.
7. Edston E, van Hage-Hamsten M, Johnasson SGO. Tryptase - at last a useful diagnostic marker for anaphylactic death. Allergy 1996:443-5.

Neutrophil Activating Peptide 2

Alaa E. Ahmed, Ph.D.

Neutrophil activating peptide-2 (NAP-2), a 75 amino acid chemokine derived from the proteolysis of beta-thromboglobulin (β-TG) by neutrophil cathepsin-G,[1-3] can activate neutrophils and monocytes by binding to their interleukin 8 (IL-8) type B receptors.[4] NAP-2 has about 60% amino acid sequence similarity with platelet factor 4 (PF-4), including a lysine-rich C-terminal α-helix that is involved in heparin binding but with lower affinity than PF-4.[4] NAP-2 is thought to augment inflammation by cooperative interactions between platelets and neutrophils.[5] Autoantibodies to NAP-2 and IL-8 are found in heparin-associated thrombocytopenia, but their clinical utility is unclear.[5] See in this Chapter: **Platelet Factor 4.**

REFERENCES
1. Gewirtz AM, Zhang J, Ratajczak J, et al. Chemokine regulation of human megakaryocytopoisis. Blood 1995;86:2559-62.
2. Car BD, Baggiolini M, Walz A. Formation of neutrophil-activating peptide 2 from platelet-derived connective-tissue-activating peptide III by different tissue proteinases. Biochem J 1991;275:581-4.
3. Waltz A, Baggiolini M. Generation of the neutrophil-activating peptide NAP-2 from platelet basic protein or connective tissue-activating peptide III through monocyte proteases. J Exp Med 1990;171:449-54.
4. Horuk R. The interleukin-8-receptor family: from chemokines to malaria. Immunol Today 1994;15:169-72.
5. Amiral J, Marfaing-Koka A, Wolf M. Presence of autoantibodies to interleukin-8 or neutrophil-activating peptide-2 in patients with heparin-associated thrombocytopenia. Blood 1996;88:410-6.

Neutrophil Nicotinamide Adenine Dinucleotide Phosphate Oxidase

E. Robert Wassman, M.D.

Defective neutrophil NADPH oxidase results in development of chronic granulomatous disease (CGD). The microbicidal activity of neutrophils depends to a large extent on the integrity of the NADPH oxidase system which, when activated, generates superoxide anion (O_2^-)and other activated oxygen species. Patients with CGD suffer from recurrent severe infections by catalase-producing organisms.[1,2] The neutrophil oxidase system is composed of a membrane-associated catalytic component and soluble cytosolic catalytic or regulatory components[2-4] encoded in chromosomal regions 1q25, 7q11.23, 16p23 and Xp21.1,[4] resulting in varying modes of inheritance. The membrane component, cytochrome b_{558}, is a heterodimer with subunits of 91 and 22 kd. Approximately 60% of patients have an X-linked form of CGD due to a mutation in the 91 kd subunit with absence of detectable cytochrome *b*. The remainder of the patients, including those with abnormal cytosolic oxidase proteins p47-phox and p67-phox and deficient cytochrome b light chain (p22-phox), manifest autosomal recessive inheritance.[4] Although exceedingly rare, dominant inheritance of CGD is described. Laboratory diagnosis is classically determined by the nitroblue tetrazolium (NBT) dye reduction test in which O_2^- reduces NBT to deep purple formazan particles.[3] In addition to being simple, widely available, and providing both qualitative and quantitative evaluation of the oxidase, the NBT test has the advantage of detecting X-linked carriers and weakly positive cell populations belonging to a variant form of CGD.[5,6] Prenatal diagnosis is possible with the NBT test using fetal blood neutrophils obtained by percutaneous umbilical blood sampling.[7] Other tests for CGD include measurements of oxygen consumption, hydrogen peroxide or O_2^- production, and chemiluminescence of phagocytes. Neutrophils can also be analyzed for the presence or absence of the different components of the NADPH oxidase system by immunoblot analysis or by flow cytometric studies.[8,9] Molecular analysis of the wide variety of specific mutations in the NADPH oxidase is possible, and forms the basis for the modern classification of CGD.[4] Deficient phagocytosis with recurrent infections can also be seen in severe G6PD deficiency, myeloperoxidase deficiency, and glutathione synthetase or reductase deficiencies.[4] See in this Chapter: **Nitroblue Tetrazolium Dye Reduction.**

REFERENCES

1. Tauber AI, Bornegaard N, Simons E, Wright J. Chronic granulomatous disease: a syndrome of phagocyte oxidase deficiencies. Medicine (Baltimore) 1983;62:286-309.
2. Volpp BD, Nauseef WM, Clark RA. Two cytosolic neutrophil oxidase components absent in autosomal chronic granulomatous disease. Science 1988;242:1295-7.
3. Smith RM, Curnutte JT. Molecular basis of chronic granulomatous disease. Blood 1991;77:673-686.
4. Forehand JR, Nauseef WM, Curnutte JT, Johnston RB. Inherited disorders of phagocyte killing. In: Scriver CR, Beaudet AL, Sly WL, Valle D, editors. The metabolic and molecular bases on inherited disease. Seventh Edition. New York: McGraw-Hill, Inc., 1995:3995-4026.
5. Baehner RL, Nathan DJ. Quantitative nitroblue tetrazolium test in chronic granulomatous disease. N Engl J Med 1968;278:971.
6. Meerhof LJ, Roos D. Heterogeneity in chronic granulomatous disease detected with an improved nitroblue tetrazolium slide test. J Leukocyte Biol 1986;39:699-711.
7. Newburger PE, Cohen HJ, Rotchild SB, et al. Prenatal diagnosis of chronic granulomatous disease. N Engl J Med 1979;300:178-9.
8. Rotrosen D, Kleinberg ME, Nuoni H, et al. Evidence of a functional domain of phagocyte oxidase cytochrome b_{558}. J Biol Chem 1990;265:8745.
9. Tsunawaki S, Mizunari H, Namiki H, Kuratsuji T. NADPH-binding component of the respiratory burst oxidase system: studies using neutrophil membranes from patients with chronic granulomatous disease lacking the β-subunit of cytochrome $b558$. J Exp Med 1994;179:291-7.

Nitroblue Tetrazolium Dye Reduction

E. Robert Wassman, M.D.

The nitroblue tetrazolium (NBT) dye reduction (NBT) is useful as a screening test for chronic granulomatous disease (CGD), a heterogeneous disorder of phagocytes in which a defective NADPH oxidase prevents production of the reactive intermediates of oxygen. This results in the failure of phagocytes to kill ingested microorganisms and predisposes patients to severe, recurrent pyogenic infections.[1-3] The nitroblue tetrazolium (NBT) dye reduction test measures the reduction of yellow soluble NBT to blue insoluble formazan by the O_2^- (superoxide) generated in intact, but stimulated (e.g., phorbol myrisate acetate [PMA] or insoluble zymosan) neutrophils.[4-6] An abnormal result should be substantiated by measurement of phagocytic bactericidal activity and quantitation of the respiratory burst by measurement of superoxide generation, chemiluminescence, oxygen consumption or hydrogen peroxide generation. Deficient phagocytosis with recurrent infections can also be seen in severe G6PD deficiency, myeloperoxidase deficiency, and glutathione synthetase or reductase deficiencies. Severe G6PD deficiency will also present a positive NBT test and a similar clinical picture, but can be distinguished by exposure to methylene blue.[7] An improvement of the classical NBT test allows use of whole blood at least 24 hours after phlebotomy employing both quantitative and qualitative assessment of NBT dye reduction. This PMA-stimulated NBT test (PMA-NBT) is useful not only for the diagnosis of CGD patients, but also for detection of carriers of CGD in X-linked CGD families when performed under conditions which reduce NBT in 100% of normal control cells.[5,6] Prenatal diagnosis is possible with the NBT test after 17 weeks of gestation; however, specific defects can also be defined by prenatal DNA analysis. Early diagnosis is of value as interferon gamma is known to decrease the frequency of infections in CGD, especially in children under 10 years of age.[8] See in this Chapter: **Neutrophil Nicotinamide Adenine Dinucleotide Phosphate Oxidase.**

REFERENCES

1. Tauber AI, Borregaard N, Simons E, Wright J. Chronic granulomatous disease: a syndrome of phagocyte oxidase deficiencies. Medicine (Baltimore) 1983;62:286-309.
2. Gallin JI, Malech HL. Update on chronic granulomatous diseases of childhood. Immunotherapy and potential for gene therapy. JAMA 1990;263:1533-7.
3. Smith RM, Curnutte JT. Molecular basis of chronic granulomatous disease. Blood 1991;77:673-86.
4. Baehner RL, Nathan DG. Quantitative nitroblue tetrazolium test in chronic granulomatous disease. N Engl J Med 1968;278:971-5.
5. Alosachie I, Peter JB, Bemiller L, Curnutte JT. An improved nitroblue tetrazolium assay for evaluation of chronic granulomatous disease. Clin Res 1991;39:438a.

6. Meerhof LJ, Roos D. Heterogeneity in chronic granulomatous disease detected with an improved nitroblue tetrazolium slide test. J Leukoc Biol 1986;39:699-711.
7. Forehand JR, Nauseef WM, Curnutte JT, Johnston RB. Inherited disorders of phagocyte killing. In: Scriver CR, Beaudet AL, Sly WL, Valle D, editors. The metabolic and molecular bases of inherited disease. Seventh Edition. New York: McGraw-Hill, Inc., 1995:3995-4026.
8. The International Chronic Granulomatous Disease Cooperative Study Group. A controlled trial of interferon gamma to prevent infection in chronic granulomatous disease. N Engl J Med 1991;324:509-16.

Nuclear Matrix Proteins

Emmanuel A. Ojo-Amaize, Ph.D.

The nuclear matrix proteins (NMPs) serve to organize the chromatin within the nucleus.[1] NMPs are associated with DNA replication, RNA synthesis, and hormone receptor binding.[1] Antibodies to NMPs react with nuclear mitotic apparatus protein (NUMA) and thus support the view that much of the nuclear matrix is used to form the mitotic apparatus (MA).[2] NMPs are linked to the cascade of cellular events that lead to programmed cell death, apoptosis.[3] Apoptosis is seen in a variety of circumstances, including immune cell selection and development,[4] ischemic or traumatic injury to the central nervous system,[5] aging,[6] cancer,[3] autoimmune states,[7] AIDS[8,9] and other pathological states. NMPs can be measured in order to analyze the effect cell death has on NUMA.[3] A sandwich enzyme immunoassay employing mouse monoclonal antibodies for measurement of soluble NMPs[3] could eventually replace methods such as MTT, ^{51}Cr, trypan blue staining,[9] ATP level, DNA fragmentation[9] and flow cytometry[8] for the measurement of apoptosis.

REFERENCES
1. Mattern KA, Humbel BM, Muijsers AO, et al. hnRNP proteins and B23 are the major proteins of the internal nuclear matrix of HeLa S3 cells. J Cell Biochem 1996;62:275-89.
2. Mancini MA, He D, Ouspenski II, Brinkley BR. Dynamic continuity of nuclear and mitotic matrix proteins in the cell cycle. J Cell Biochem 1996;62:158-64.
3. Miller T, Beausang LA, Meneghini M, Lidgard G. Death-induced changes to the nuclear matrix: the use of anti-nuclear matrix antibodies to study agents of apoptosis. Biotechniques 1993;15:1042-7.
4. Majno G, Joris J. Apoptosis, oncosis and necrosis: an overview of cell death. Am J Pathol 1995;146:3-15.
5. Johnson EM, Greenlund LJ, Hsu CY. Neuronal apoptososis: current understanding of molecular mechanisms and potential role in ischemic brain injury. J Neurotrauma 1995;5:843-52.
6. Dell'Orco RT, Whittle WL. Nuclear matrix composition and in vitro cellular senescence. Exp Gerontol 1994;29:139-49.
7. Zuber M, Heyden TS, Lajous-Petter AM. A human autoantibody recognizing nuclear matrix-associated nuclear protein localized in dot structures. Biol Cell 1995;85:77-86.
8. Glynn JM, McElligott DL, Mosier DE. Apoptosis induced by HIV infection in H9 T cells is blocked by ICE-family protease inhibition but nor by a Fas (CD95) antagonists. J Immunol 1996;157:2754-8.
9. Gronx H, Torpier G, Monte D, et al. Activation-induced death by apoptosis in CD4$^+$ T cells from human immunodeficiency virus-infected asymptomatic individuals. J Exp Med 1992;175:331-40.

Phagocyte Disorders

Paula D'Amore, Ph.D.

Phagocytic disorders are characterized by recurrent bacterial infections that can involve the skin, respiratory tract and lymph nodes. In more severe cases, infections can be systemic and sometimes fatal. Specific tests for phagocytic disorders should be considered only after testing of humoral and cellular function has been evaluated.

An evaluation of phagocytosis should include the following tests:

	Tests	Comments
Motility	Capillary tube method	Purified neutrophils in a microhematocrit tube. Random motility is assessed.

	Tests	Comments
	Rebuck skin window	*In vivo* evaluation of neutrophil motility, rarely used.
Chemotaxis	Radical migration	Wells cut in agarose medium. Chemo-attractants placed in one well and neutrophils in the other. Chemotactic migration of neutrophils is assessed. Defective in leukocyte adhesion deficiency, Chediak-Higashi syndrome, Job syndrome.
Adhesion	Flow cytometry CD11a CD11b CD11c CD18	Membrane glycoprotein (integrins) present on neutrophils, monocytes, and some lymphoctes. Function as adhesion molecules. Deficient in leukocyte adhesion.
Intracellular killing (Respiratory burst)	1. Nitroblue tetrazolium dye reduction test 2. Chemiluminescence	Defects related to oxidative burst and superoxide generation. Abnormal in chronic granulomatous disease (CGD), myeloperoxidase deficiency.
Enzyme testing	Myeloperoxidase	MPO deficiency
Peripheral blood smear	Giant cytoplasmic Granular inclusions in leukocytes	Chediak-Higashi syndrome

Chronic granulomatous disease: Chronic granulomatous disease (CDG) is an inherited, X-linked disorder characterized by recurrent infections in the lungs, skin, lymph nodes and intestinal tract. The infections are normally associated with low virulent organisms such as *Staphylococcus epidermis* and *Serratia marcescans*.

The respiratory burst in the neutrophils is deficient due to a defect in one of the components of the nicotinamide adenine dinucleotides phosphate oxidase (NADPH) system.[1] Reflecting the inability to generate superoxide (O_2^-), hydrogen peroxide (H_2O_2) and hypochlorite (OCL^-), the neutrophils are unable to kill microorganisms. The primary tests available for diagnosis are the NBT and chemiluminescence.

Myeloperoxidase deficiency: Myeloperoxidase (MPO) is necessary for intracellular killing of certain organisms by neutrophils and monocytes. A complete or partial deficiency of MPO can occur in this inherited disorder.[2] The respiratory burst is mildly prolonged. Susceptibility to *Candida* and *Staphylococcus* infections is a major consequence. Diagnosis is established by demonstrating an MPO deficiency in the neutrophils and monocytes.

Job syndrome (Hyperimmunoglobulin E syndrome): Job syndrome is characterized by recurrent cold abscesses of the skin and sinopulmonary tract. The organisms involved most often include *Staphylococcus aureus*, *Streptococcus pneumoniae*, group A strep and *Candida*. A hyper IgE response against *S. aureus* and defective chemotaxis are diagnostic.[3]

Chediak-Higashi syndrome: Chediak-Higashi syndrome is an autosomal recessive disorder of recurrent bacterial infections, partial albinism, and hepatosplenomegaly. A high incidence of lymphoreticular malignacies are common in patients surviving the first decade of life. Giant cytoplasmic inclusions, formed by the fusion of granules, are seen in all blood cells. Abnormal microtubule function and increased levels of cyclic AMP (cAMP) contribute to the impaired neutrophil chemotaxis. Increased EBV antibody titers, decreased natural killer (NK) cell activity, and antibody-dependent cell-mediated cytotoxicity are also common.[3]

Leukocyte adhesion deficiency: Individuals with leukocyte adhesion deficiency (LAD) have impaired leukocyte adhesion and chemotaxis resulting in recurrent pyogenic infections and an inability to form pus. Delayed separation of the umbilical cord is also seen. Three cell surface integrins (CD11a, CD11b, CD11c) are not expressed.[4] All three have distinct α-chains and a common β-chain (CD18). There is a deficiency in the β-chain which is responsible for the lack of expression of CD11a, CD11b, and CD11c. These result in the phagocyte's inability to adhere strongly to the vascular endothelial cells, thus eliminating the emigration of the phagocytic cell between the endothelial cells and migration to the inflammatory stimuli.[5] Because the leukocytes lack the CD11b/CD18 integrin (receptor for the C_3bi complement fragment), they are unable to bind opsonized microrganisms.[6] Decreased neutrophil chemotaxis and adhesion are diagnostic of LAD I. In LAD II there is an absence of the siayl-Lewis X ligand of ε-selectin.[7,8]

Miscellaneous phagocytic disorders: Numerous rare phagocytic disorders exist and include deficiencies of specific granules (i.e., lactoferrin) or other secondary granules resulting in decreased chemotaxis and little bactericidal activity.[9]

Secondary neutrophil dysfunction: Various disorders such as acute non-lymphocytic leukemia, myeloproliferative, myelodysplastic and lymphoproliferative syndromes can lead to a secondary neutrophil function defect. See in this Chapter: **Leukocyte Adhesion Molecules.**

REFERENCES

1. Curnutte JT. Chronic granulomatous disease: the solving of a clinical riddle at the molecular level. Clin Immunol Immunopathol 1993;67:S2-S15.
2. Nauseel WM. Myeloperoxidase deficiency. Hematol Pathol 1990;4:165-78.
3. Nagle DL, Karim MA, Woolf EA, et al. Identification and mutation analysis of the complete gene for Chediak-Higashi syndrome. Nat Genet 1996;14:307-11.
4. Harlan JM. Leukocyte adhesion deficiency syndrome: insights into the molecular basis of leukocyte emigration. Clin Immunol Immunopathol 1993;67:S16-S24.
5. Stickle JE. The neutrophil: function, disorders and testing. Vet Clin North Am 1996;5:1013-21.
6. Bevilacqua MP. Endothelial-leukocyte adhesion molecules. Annu Rev Immunol 1993;11:767-84.
7. Etzioni A, Frydmam M, Pollack S, et al. Recurrent infections caused by a novel leukocyte adhesion deficiency. N Engl J Med 1992;327:1789-92.
8. Etzioni A. Adhesion molecules - - their role in health and disease. Pediatr Res 1996;39:191-8.
9. Moretti S, Lanza F, Spisani S, et al. Neutrophils from patients with myelodysplastic syndromes: relationship between impairement of granular contents, complement receptors, functional activities and disease status. Leuk Lymphoma 1994;13:471-7.

Plasma Histamine

Sonny Gunawan, Ph.D.

Although release of histamine from basophils and mast cells is an important step in most immediate hypersensitivity reactions,[1] and commercial RIA and EIA kits[2] as well as HPLC assay[3] are available, plasma histamine determinations are rarely utilized in the evaluation of allergic patients. This is due in large measure to the short half-life of histamine in plasma, which makes time-course studies essential.[4] Plasma histamine measurements can be used to establish and to separate acute- and late-phase reactions, but mast cell tryptase and thromboxane A_2[5] are the preferred analytes due to their longer half-life. See Chapter 6: **Thromboxane A₂.**

REFERENCES

1. Sampson HA, Jolie PL. Increased plasma histamine concentrations after food challenges in children with atopic dermatitis. N Engl J Med 1984;311:372-6.
2. Ownby DR. *In vitro* assays for the evaluation of immunologic reactions to foods. Immunol Allergy Clin North Am 1991;11:851-62.

3. Kumura K, Hirai E, Uchida K, Kikuchi J, Terui Y. Quantification of histamine by postcolumn fluorescence detection high-performance liquid chromatography using orthophthalaldehyde in tetrahydrofuran and reaction mechanism. Anal Sci 1994;10:259-65.
4. Schwartz LB, Yunginger JW, Miller J, Bokhari R, Dull D. Time course of appearance and disappearance of human mast cell tryptase in the circulation after anaphylaxis. J Clin Invest 1989;83:1551-5.
5. Ohtsuka T, Matsumaru S, Uchida K, et al. Pathogenic role of thromboxane A_2 in immediate food hypersensitivity reactions in children. Ann Allergy Asthma Immunol 1996;77:55-9.

Platelet Factor 4

Alaa E. Ahmed, Ph.D.

Platelet factor 4, a chemokine which is a major constituent of platelet alpha granules, has sequence similarities to both beta-thromboglobulin (βTG) and neutrophil activating peptide-2 (NAP-2).[1,2] PAF is an asymmetrically associated homo-tetrameric protein (70 residues/subunit) known for binding polysulfated glycosaminoglycans such as heparin.[3]

Various activities documented for PF4 include: heparin binding, which neutralizes the anti-thrombin activity of anti-thrombin III (AT-III); inhibition of angiogenesis; induction of ICAM-1 on endothelial cells; promotion of neutrophil adhesion to endothelium; increased fibrin fiber formation; inhibition of other chemotactic factor effects; *in vivo* recruitment of neutrophils; fibroblast migration during wound repair; and reversal of Con-A-induced suppression of lymphocyte activity.[4] Complexes of PAF and heparin are the targets for heparin induced autoantibodies (HIT).[5] See in this Chapter: **Neutrophil Activating Peptide 2**.

REFERENCES
1. Zucker MB, Katz IR. Platelet factor 4: production, structure and physiologic and immunologic action. Proc Soc Exp Biol Med 1991;198:693-702.
2. Car BD, Baggiolini M, Walz A. Formation of neutrophil-activating peptide 2 from platelet-derived connective- tissue-activating peptide III by different tissue proteinases. Biochem J 1991;275:581-4.
3. Mayo KH, Ilyina E, Roongta V, et al. Heparin binding to platelet factor-4. An NMR and site-directed mutagenesis study. Biochem J 1995;1:357-65.
4. Engstad CS, Lia K, Rekdal O, et al. A novel biological effect of platelet factor-4 (PF4): enhancement of LPS-induced tissue factor activity in monocytes. J Leukoc Biol 1995;58:575-81.
5. Arepally G, Cines DB. Heparin-associated autoantibodies. In: Peter JB, Shoenfeld Y, editors. Autoantibodies. Amsterdam: Elsevier Science B.V., 1996:343-50.

Chapter 4
Bacterial and Fungal
Hypersensitivity Reactions

Alternaria spp.

Herminio R. Reyes, Ph.D.

The most important class of aeroallergenic fungi is *Deuteromycetes* which includes *Alternaria*, *Cladosporium*, *Penicillium*, *Aspergillus* and *Phoma* spp.[1] Many of these fungi can induce hypersensitivity pneumonitis (HP).[2,3] *Alternaria* spp. cause hypersensitivity pneumonitis (HP) known as woodworker's lung disease,[4] as well as IgE-mediated allergic disease, which is very common in individuals with atopic disease.[1]

RAST and immunoblot analysis using standardized, partially purified *A. tenuis* antigens detect *Alternaria*-specific IgE in over 94% of children with a positive bronchial provocation test (BPT) to *A. tenuis*, but immunoblot analysis also detects IgE to *Cladosporium* spp. in most of these children.[5] Differential diagnosis of allergy due to *A. tenuis* and *Cladosporium herbarum* is difficult, because many individuals can have simultaneous allergies to both fungi.[5] Cross-reactivity of *A. tenuis* with *C. herbarum*, as well as *Aspergillus fumigatus*, is evident from immunoblot analysis and RAST.[6] IgE against *Alternaria* spp. is also detected in some nonallergic children, although the immunoblot bands are fewer and less intense than those from allergic children.[5] False-positives in nonallergic individuals are probably due to the ubiquitous nature of *Alternaria* spp. in the environment.[5] Therefore, in addition to IgE reactivity, patient history and symptoms must be considered in making an accurate diagnosis of IgE-mediated allergy to *Alternaria* spp.[5] *Alternaria* spp. also cause cutaneous phaeohyphomycosis.[7] See in this Chapter: *Aspergillus* **spp.**, *Cladosporium* **spp.**, *Penicillium* **spp.** and *Phoma* **spp.**

REFERENCES
1. Salvaggio J, Aukrust L. Mold-induced asthma. J Allergy Clin Immunol 1981;68:327-46.
2. Levy MB, Fink JN. Hypersensitivity pneumonitis. Ann Allergy 1985;54:167-72.
3. Escudero AI, Sanchez-Guerrero IM, Mora AM, et al. Cost-effectiveness of various methods of diagnosing hypersensitivity to Alternaria. Allergol Immunopathol 1993;21:153-7.
4. Sosman AJ, Schlueter DP, Fink JN, Barboriak JJ. Hypersensitivity to wood dust. N Engl J Med 1969;281:977-80.
5. Nusslein HG, Zimmermann T, Baum M, et al. Improved in vitro diagnosis of allergy to *Alternaria tenius* and *Cladosporium herbarum*. Allergy 1987;42:414-22.
6. Tee RD, Gordon DJ, Taylor AJ. Cross-reactivity between antigens of fungal extracts studied by RAST inhibition and immunoblot technique. J Allergy Clin Immunol 1987;79:627-33.
7. Ajello L. Hyalohyphomycosis and phaeohyphomycosis: two global disease entities of public health importance. Eur J Epidemiol 1986;2:243-51.

Aspergillus spp.

Herminio R. Reyes, Ph.D.

The most important class of aeroallergenic fungi is *Deuteromycetes* which includes *Aspergillus*, *Alternaria*, *Cladosporium*, *Penicillium* and *Phoma* spp.;[1] many of these fungi can induce hypersensitivity pneumonitis (HP).[2] *Aspergillus* spp. together with the thermophilic actinomyces, including *Thermoactinomyces vulgaris* and *Faenia rectivirgula* (*Micropolyspora faeni*), are the most common causes of the HP known as farmer's lung disease.[3] Other types of HP caused by *Aspergillus* spp. are malt worker's (*A. fumigatus* and *A. clavatus*),[4] tobacco worker's [5] and compost lung diseases.[6]

Aspergillus spp. also cause three distinct illnesses, including allergic bronchopulmonary aspergillosis (ABPA), pulmonary aspergilloma (fungus ball) and invasive aspergillosis (IA).[7] IA is the most difficult to diagnose, is most common in AIDS and otherwise immunocompromised patients and is often fatal.[7-9] ABPA, a type of eosinophilic pneumonia, is sometimes confused with HP because of the presence of precipitating antibodies to *A. fumigatus*.[10] ABPA occurs in about 1-2% of patients with chronic asthma; use of appropriate positive and negative controls are important for differential diagnosis.[11,12] For the diagnosis of ABPA and aspergilloma, EIA and ID are the most frequently used assays and have sensitivities of 93% and 64% and specificities of 89% and 100%, respectively, using *A. fumigatus* antigens in culture-proven cases.[13] EIA and LA sensitivities of 90% and 70% and specificities of 84% and 86% are reported for IA in chemotherapy-induced neutropenia.[14] The sensitivity of LA is too low for diagnosis of early IA, but might be useful when cultures remain negative and serial specimens are tested.[15] The sensitivity of ID can be improved by use of concentrated sera, but weak positive results to only one extract should be interpreted with caution in patients without clinical evidence of mycetoma or ABPA.[16] EIA is more rapid than ID and allows direct measurement of IgG, IgM, IgA and IgE antibodies;[11-13,17] positive EIA results should be confirmed by immunoblotting.[18] ABPA patients are monitored by measuring total serum IgE; a two-fold increase can indicate the prodrome of an exacerbation.[19]

The antibody response to *A. fumigatus* antigens is polyclonal;[20] rises in serum levels of *A. fumigatus*-specific IgG, IgA and IgM with disease activity are reported.[13,21] *Alternaria tenuis* and *Cladosporium herbarum* cross-react with *A. fumigatus* in immunoblot analysis and in RAST of sera from patients with IgE-mediated allergic disease.[22] IgG and IgE antibodies to low molecular weight *A. fumigatus* antigens are found consistently in sera from ABPA patients by immunoblot analysis[23] and by RAST in cystic fibrosis patients.[24] *A. fumigatus*-specific IgE and IgG antibodies can also be detected by crossed radioimmunoelectrophoresis (CRIE) in sera of patients with aspergilloma, ABPA and extrinsic asthma with *Aspergillus* allergy.[25]

In aspergilloma, *A. fumigatus*-specific IgE and elevated total IgE are not usually detected, but high levels of IgG antibodies are diagnostically useful.[7,23,26] When ABPA complicates aspergilloma, however, high levels of both total and *A. fumigatus*-specific IgE are detected.[7,26] Antibodies reactive with high molecular weight *A. fumigatus* antigens are found frequently in sera from patients with aspergilloma by immunoblot analysis.[23] For diagnosis of IA, EIA is 84% sensitive for the detection of IgG reactive with somatic or culture filtrate antigens of *A. fumigatus*.[27] Reactivity with somatic antigens is useful in early disseminated disease; whereas, culture filtrate antigens give the best overall sensitivity.[27] Prospective study of patients who will be immunosuppressed is often useful to document presence of antibody because antibodies can disappear by the time IA is diagnosed.[27] Studies utilizing isoelectric focusing with immunoblotting suggest that using a spectrum of antigens is advisable for antibody detection because of great variability in immune responses between individuals.[28]

Assays for detection of antigenemia show variable sensitivity (17–75%), probably due to the rapid clearance of *Aspergillus* galactomannan,[29] but are quite specific (94–100%).[30-33] Antigenemia correlates with extent of infection in IA.[34] False-positives with LA tests can occur which might result from instability of sera during storage or less than optimal test conditions.[35,36] IB[37] and EIA[38] analysis of urine from patients with IA detects galactomannan and non-galactomannan antigens of *Aspergillus* spp.[29,37] Purification and characterization of these antigens, as well as recombinant antigens,[39,40] should lead to more sensitive and specific immunoassays[41,42] with positive and negative predictive values approaching 100%.[38] A 100 kd band on IB analysis of CSF is a potential marker for poor outcome in patients with central nervous system aspergillosis.[43] Murine monoclonal antibodies produced against components of *A. fumigatus* antigens[44] associated with ABPA[45] should also improve sensitivity and specificity of immunoassays. The antigenic components reactive with some monoclonals are mostly of low molecular weight and also react with IgG and IgE in sera from patients with ABPA but not with aspergilloma.[45] Studies of the interactions of *A. fumigatus* proteins with complement components should clarify the role of alternate complement pathway activation in *Aspergillus* infections.[46]

Defects in phagocytic host defenses against *Aspergillus* may contribute to development of invasive aspergillosis in HIV-infected patients without other predisposing factors.[47] A comprehensive review of the characteristic features of *Aspergillus*-induced diseases and the immunology, etiology, epidemiology and immunodiagnosis of aspergillosis is available.[48] Molecular detection and typing methods including PCR are promising for rapid diagnosis and epidemiologic studies.[49-55] See in this Chapter: ***Alternaria* spp.**, ***Cladosporium* spp.**, ***Faenia rectivirgula*, *Penicillium* spp.**, ***Phoma* spp.** and ***Thermoactinomyces* spp.**

REFERENCES

1. Salvaggio J, Aukrust L. Mold-induced asthma. J Allergy Clin Immunol 1981;68:327-46.
2. Levy MB, Fink JN. Hypersensitivity pneumonitis. Ann Allergy 1985;54:167-72.
3. Pepys J, Jenkins PA. Farmer's lung. Thermophilic actinomycetes as a source of "farmer's lung hay" antigen. Lancet 1963;2:607-11.
4. Channell S, Blyth W, Lloyd M, et al. Allergic alveolitis in maltworkers. A clinical, mycological, and immunological study. Q J Med 1969;38:351-76.
5. Huuskonen MS, Husman K, Jarvisalo J, et al. Extrinsic allergic alveolitis in the tobacco industry. Br J Ind Med 1984;41:77-83.
6. Vincken W, Roels P. Hypersensitivity pneumonitis due to Aspergillus fumigatus. Thorax 1984;39:74-5.
7. Boon AP, O'Brien D, Adams DH. 10 year review of invasive aspergillosis detected at necropsy. J Clin Pathol 1991;44:452-4.
8. Denning DW, Follansbee SE, Scolaro M, Norris S, Edelstein H, Stevens DA. Pulmonary aspergillosis in the acquired immunodeficiency syndrome. N Engl J Med 1991;324:654-62.
9. Hovenden JL, Nicklason F, Barnes RA. Invasive pulmonary aspergillosis in non-immunocompromised patients. Br Med J 1991;302:583-4.
10. Richerson HB, Bernstein IL, Fink JN, et al. Guidelines for the clinical evaluation of hypersensitivity pneumonitis. J Allergy Clin Immunol 1989;84(5 Pt 2):839-44.
11. Bernstein JA, Zeiss CR, Greenberger PA, Patterson R, Marhoul JF, Smith LL. Immunoblot analysis of sera from patients with allergic bronchopulmonary aspergillosis: correlation with disease activity. J Allergy Clin Immunol 1990;86:532-9.
12. Hutcheson PS, Rejent AJ Slavin RG. Variability in parameters of allergic bronchopulmonary aspergillosis in patients with cystic fibrosis. J Allergy Clin Immunol 1991;88:390-4.
13. Froudist JH, Harnett GB, McAleer R. Comparison of immunodiffusion and enzyme linked immunosorbent assay for antibodies to four Aspergillus species. J Clin Pathol 1989;42:1215-21.
14. Verweij PE, Stynen D, Rijs AJMM, De Pauw BE, Hoogkamp-Korstanje JAA, Meis JFGM. Sandwich enzyme-linked immunosorbent assay compared with Pastorex latex agglutination test for diagnosing invasive aspergillosis in immunocompromised patients. J Clin Microbiol 1995;33:1912-4.
15. Verweij PE, Rijs AJ, De Pauw BE, et al. Clinical evaluation and reproducibility of the Pastorex Aspergillus antigen latex agglutination test for diagnosing invasive aspergillosis. J Clin Pathol 1995;48:474-6.
16. Faux JA, Shale DJ, Lane DJ. Precipitins and specific IgG antibody to Aspergillus fumigatus in a chest unit population. Thorax 1992:47:48-52.
17. Knutsen Ap, Hutcheson PS, Mueller KR, Slavin RG. Serum immunoglobulins E and G anti-Aspergillus fumigatus antibody in patients with cystic fibrosis who have allergic bronchopulmonary aspergillosis. J Lab Clin Med 1990;116:724-7.
18. Brouwer J. Detection of antibodies against Aspergillus fumigatus: comparison between double immunodiffusion, ELISA and immunoblot analysis. Int Arch Allergy Appl Immunol 1988;85:244-9.
19. Greenberger PA. Allergic bronchopulmonary aspergillosis and fungoses. Clin Chest Med 1988;9:599-608.
20. Ojanen T. Class specific antibodies in serodiagnosis of farmer's lung. Br J Indus Med 1992;49:332-6.
21. Apter AJ, Greenberger PA, Liotta JL, Roberts M. Fluctuations of serum IgA and its subclasses in allergic bronchopulmonary aspergillosis. J Allergy Clin Immunol 1989;84:367-72.
22. Tee RD, Gordon DJ, Taylor AJ. Cross-reactivity between antigens of fungal extracts studied by RAST inhibition and immunoblot technique. J Allergy Clin Immunol 1987;79:627-33.
23. Kurup VP, Greenberger PA, Fink JN. Antibody response to low-molecular-weight antigens of Aspergillus fumigatus in allergic bronchopulmonary aspergillosis. J Clin Microbiol 1989;27:1312-6.
24. El-Dahr JM, Fink R, Selden R, Arruda LK, Platts-Mills TAE, Heymann PW. Development of immune responses to Aspergillus at an early age in children with cystic fibrosis. Am J Respir Crit Care Med 1994;150:1513-8.
25. Wallenbeck I, Dreborg S, Zetterström, Einarsson R. Aspergillus fumigatus-specific IgE and IgG antibodies for diagnosis of Aspergillus-related lung diseases. Allergy 1991;46:372-8.

26. Anderson CJ, Craig S, Bardana Jr EJ. Allergic bronchopulmonary aspergilliosis and bilateral fungal balls terminating in disseminated aspergillosis. J Allergy Clin Immunol 1980;65:140-4.
27. Trull AK, Parker J, Warren RE. IgG enzyme linked immunosorbent assay for diagnosis of invasive aspergillosis: retrospective study over 15 years of transplant recipients. J Clin Pathol 1985;38:1045-51.
28. Hearn VM, Pinel C, Blachier S, Ambroise-Thomas P, Grillot R. Specific antibody detection in invasive aspergillosis by analytical isoelctrofocusing and immunoblotting methods. J Clin Microbiol 1995;33:982-6.
29. de Repentigny L. Serodiagnosis of candidiasis, aspergillosis, and cryptococcosis. Clin Infect Dis 1992;14:S11-22.
30. Weiner MH, Talbot GH, Gerson SL, Filice G, Cassileth PA. Antigen detection in the diagnosis of invasive aspergilosis. Ann Intern Med 1983;99:777-82.
31. Sabetta JR, Miniter P, Andriole VT. The diagnosis of invasive aspergillosis by an enzyme-linked immunosorbent assay for circulating antigen. J Infect Dis 1985;152:946-53.
32. Dupont B, Huber M, Kim SJ, Bennett JE. Galactomannan antigenemia and antigenuria is aspergillosis: studies in patients and experimentally infected rabbits. J Infect Dis 1987;155:1-11.
33. Manso E, Montillo M, de Sio G, D'Amico S, Discepoli G, Leoni P. Value of antigen and antibody detection in the serological diagnosis of invasive aspergillosis in patients with hematological malignancies. Eur J Clin Microbiol Infect Dis 1994;13:756-60.
34. Patterson TF, Miniter P, Patterson JE, Rappeport JM, Andriole VT. *Aspergillus* antigen detection in the diagnosis of invasive aspergillosis. J Infect Dis 1995;171;1553-8.
35. Warnock DW, Foot ABM, Johnson EM, Mitchell SB, Cornish JM, Oakhill A. *Aspergillus* antigen latex test for diagnosis of invasive aspergillosis [Letter]. Lancet 1991;338:1023-4.
36. Knight F, Mackenzie DWR, Stynen D, Meulemans L, Garrigues ML. *Aspergillus* antigen latex test for diagnosis of invasive aspergillosis [Letters]. Lancet 1992;339:188.
37. Haynes KA, Latge JP, Rogers TR. Detection of *Aspergillus* antigens associated with invasive infection. J Clin Microbiol 1990;28:2040-4.
38. Rogers TR, Haynes KA, Barnes RA. Value of antigen detection in predicting invasive pulmonary aspergillosis. Lancet 1990;336:1210-3.
39. Moser M, Crameri R, Brust E, Suter M, Menz G. Diagnostic value or recombinant Aspergillus fumigatus allergen I/a for skin testing and serology. J Allergy Clin Immunol 1994;93:1-11.
40. Disch R, Menz G, Blaser K, Crameri R. Different reactivity to recombinant *Aspergillus fumigatus* allergen I/a in patients with atopic dermatitis or allergic asthma sensitised to *Aspergillus fumigatus*. Int Arch Allergy Immunol 1995;108:89-94.
41. de Repentigny L, Kilanowski E, Pedneault L, Boushira M. Immunoblot analyses of the serologic response to *Aspergillus fumigans* antigens in experimental invasive aspergillosis. J Infect Dis 1991;163:1305-11.
42. Lopez-Medrano R, Ovejero MC, Calera JA, Puente P, Leal F. Aspergillus fumigatus antigens. Microbiology 1995;141:2699-704.
43. Ray P, Chakrabarti A, Jatana M, Sharma BS, Pathak A. Western blot analysis of cerebrospinal fluid for detection of *Aspergillus* antigens. Mycopathologica 1995;131:103-6.
44. Ste-Marie L, Sénéchal S, Boushira M, et al. Production and characterization of monoclonal antibodies to cell wall antigens of Aspergillus fumigatus. Infect Immun 1990;58:2105-14.
45. Kurup VP. Murine monoclonal antibodies binding to the specific antigens of *Aspergillus fumigatus* associated with allergic bronchopulmonary aspergillosis. J Clin Lab Anal 1989;3:116-21.
46. Sturtevant JE, Latge J-P. Interactions between conidia of *Aspergillus fumigatus* and human complement component C3. Infect Immun 1992;60:1913-8.
47. Roilides E, Holmes A, Blake C, Pizzo PA, Walsh TJ. Defective antifungal activity of monocyte-derived macrophages from human immunodeficiency virus-infected children against *Aspergillus fumigatus*. J Infect Dis 1993;168:1562-5.
48. Kurup VP, Kumar A. Immunodiagnosis of aspergillosis. Clin Microbiol Rev 1991;4:439-56.
49. Pfaller MA. Epidemiology of fungal infections: the promise of molecular typing. Clin Infect Dis 1995;20:1535-9.
50. Bretagne S, Costa JM, Marmorat-Khuong A, et al. Detection of *Aspergillus* species DNA in bronchoalveolar lavage samples by competitive PCR. J Clin Microbiol 1995;33:1164-8.
51. Verweij PE, Latgé J-P, Rijs AJMM, et al. Comparison of antigen detection and PCR assay using bronchoalveolar lavage fluid for diagnosing invasive pulmonary aspergillosis in patients receiving treatment for hematological malignancies. J Clin Microbiol 1995;33:3150-3.
52. Melchers WJG, Verweij PE, van den Hurk P, et al. General primer-mediated PCR for detection of Aspergillus species. J Clin Microbiol 1994;32:1710-7.
53. Makimura K, Murayama SY, Yamaguchi H. Specific detection of *Aspergillus* and *Penicillium* species from respiratory specimens by polymerase chain reaction (PCR). Jpn J Med Sci Biol 1994;47:141-56.

54. Loudon KW, Burnie JP, Coke AP, Matthews RC. Application of polymerase chain reaction to fingerprinting *Aspergillus fumigatus* by random amplification of polymorphic DNA. J Clin Microbiol 1993;31:1117-21.

55. Rinyu E, Varga J, Ferenczy L. Phenotypic and genotypic analysis of variability in *Aspergillus fumigatus*. J Clin Microbiol 1995;33:2567-75.

Cladosporium spp.

Herminio R. Reyes, Ph.D.

The most important class of aeroallergenic fungi is *Deuteromycetes* which includes *Alternaria*, *Cladosporium*, *Penicillium*, *Aspergillus* and *Phoma* spp.;[1] many of these fungi can induce hypersensitivity pneumonitis (HP).[2] *Cladosporium* spp. causes HP known as hot tub lung disease,[3] as well as IgE-mediated allergic disease, which is very common in individuals with atopic disease.[1]

An accurate diagnosis of allergy to *Cladosporium* spp. can be made based on asthma symptoms which follow the seasonal variations in the *Cladosporium* spore counts and the demonstration of IgE reactivity, including an unequivocally positive bronchial provocation test (BPT);[4] false-positive BPTs, however, can occur in asthmas due to other causes.[5,6] For detection of IgE reactivity, the skin prick test using purified, characterized and potent (100,000 biological units) extract of *C. herbarum* is recommended as a primary screening test because it is rarely false-negative; RAST, crossed- radioimmunoelectrophoresis and histamine release from basophil granulocytes can be negative in 20-30% of patients with positive allergy.[4,7] RAST using purified, characterized extracts is optimal to confirm the presence of *Cladosporium*-specific IgE because it is rarely false-positive.[4] Differential diagnosis of allergy due to *C. herbarum* and *Alternaria tenuis* can be difficult, however, because many individuals can have simultaneous allergies to both fungi;[7] cross-reactivity of *C. herbarum* with *A. tenuis* as well as with *Aspergillus fumigatus* is evident from immunoblot analysis and RAST of sera.[8] The degree of IgE reactivity to *Cladosporium* is not predictive of the severity of the allergy.[4]

Although microscopy is the most rapid and reliable method for diagnosis of chromoblastomycosis due to *C. carrionii*, it is not useful for evaluating prognosis or response to therapy.[9] ID and counterimmunoelectrophoresis (CIE) detect antibodies to *C. carrionii* in sera of most (>85%) patients with chromoblastomycosis due to *C. carrionii*; CIE is more rapid than ID.[9,10] The use of culture filtrate antigens from *C. carrionii* in ID and CIE allows differentiation of *C. carrionii* from *Phialophora verrucosa* and prevents cross-reactions with *Fonsecaea pedrosoi*, the other etiologic agents of chromoblastomycosis.[11,12] Recombinant allergens will be useful for characterization and standardization of allergenic extracts.[13,14]

Phaeohyphomycosis due to *C. trichoides* and *C. bantianum* (*Xylohypha bantiana*) occurs worldwide, predominantly in young males, and usually affects the CNS;[15-17] immunosuppression can be a predisposing factor for development of this disease.[18] See in this Chapter: *Alternaria* spp., *Aspergillus* spp., *Penicillium* spp. and *Phoma* spp.

REFERENCES

1. Salvaggio J, Aukrust L. Mold-induced asthma. J Allergy Clin Immunol 1981;68:327-46.
2. Levy MB, Fink JN. Hypersensitivity pneumonitis. Ann Allergy 1985;54:167-72.
3. Jacobs RL, Thorner RE, Holcomb JR, Schwietz LA, Jacobs FO. Hypersensitivity pneumonitis caused by Cladosporium in an enclosed hot-tub area. Ann Intern Med 1986;105:204-6.
4. Malling H-J. Diagnosis and immunotherapy of mould allergy. Danish Med Bull 1990;37:12-22.
5. Aas K. Heterogeneity of bronchial asthma. Sub-populations - or different stages of the disease. Allergy 1981;36:3-14.
6. Nelson NS. Diagnostic procedures in allergy. II. Bronchial provocation testing. Ann Allergy 1983;51:488-92.
7. Nusslein HG, Zimmermann T, Baum M, et al. Improved in vitro diagnosis of allergy to *Alternaria tenius* and *Cladosporium herbarum*. Allergy 1987;42:414-22.

8. Tee RD, Gordon DJ, Taylor AJ. Cross-reactivity between antigens of fungal extracts studied by RAST inhibition and immunoblot technique. J Allergy Clin Immunol 1987;79:627-33.

9. Villalba E. Detection of antibodies in the sera of patients with chromboblastomycosis by counter immunoelectrophoresis I. Preliminary results. J Med Vet Mycol 1988;26:73-4.

10. Villalba E, Yegres JF. Detection of circulating antibodies in patients affected by chromoblastomycosis by Cladosporium carrionii using double immunodiffusion. Mycopathologia 1988;102:17-9.

11. Cooper BH, Schneidau JD. A serological comparison of *Phialophora verrucosa*, *Fonsecaea pedrosoi* and *Cladosporium carrinii* using immunodiffusion and immunoelectrophoresis. Sabouraudia 1970;8:217-26.

12. Nicolaisen L, Swatek FE. Some studies of exoantigens for the identification of the causative agents of chromoblastomycosis. In: Proceedings of the Fifth International Conference on the Mycoses. Medellin: Pan American Health Organization, 1980:259-64.

13. Achantz G, Oberkofler H, Lechenauer E, et al. Molecular cloning of major and minor allergens of *Alternaria alternata* and *Cladosporium herbarum*. Mol Immunol 1995;32:213-27.

14. Zhang L, Muradia G, Curran IH, Rode H, Vijay HM. A cDNA clone coding for a novel allergen, Cla h III, of *Cladosporium herbarum* identified as a ribosomal P2 protein. J Immunol 1995;154:710-7.

15. Nadkarni TD, Goel A, Shenoy A, Karapurkar AP. *Cladosporium bantianum* (*trichoides*) infection of the brain. J Postgrad Med 1993;39:43-4.

16. Palaoglu S, Sav A, Basak T, Yalcinlar Y, Scheithauer BW. Cerebral phaeohyphomycosis. Neurosurgery 1993;33:894-7.

17. Sekhon AS, Galbraith J, Mielke BW, Garg AK, Sheehan G. Cerebral phaeohyphomycosis caused by *Xylohypha bantiana*, with a review of the literature. Eur J Epidemiol 1992;8:387-90.

18. Aldape KD, Fox HS, Roberts JP, Ascher NL, Lake JR, Rowley HA. *Cladosporium trichoides* cerebral phaeohyphomycosis in a liver transplant recipient. Am J Clin Pathol 1991;95:499-502.

Faenia rectivirgula

Herminio R. Reyes, Ph.D.

Faenia rectivirgula, previously known as *Micropolyspora faeni*,[1] is the most frequently incriminated inhalant in farmer's lung disease, the most common hypersensitivity pneumonitis (HP) in the United States.[2-5] *F. rectivirgula*, or antigens thereof, stimulate IL-1 production by human alveolar macrophages and high-level secretion of tumor necrosis factor-α (TNF-α) from human alveolar macrophages and monocytes, implicating direct stimulation of cytokine release in the pathogenesis of HP.[6] Precipitin antibodies (more commonly reactive with *F. rectivirgula* than with other thermophilic actinomycetes) are found in 10–20% of exposed, asymptomatic individuals.[3] *F. rectivirgula*-reactive antibodies of IgG, IgM, IgA and IgE classes are commonly found in symptomatic and in unaffected subjects.[2,7] *F. rectivirgula*-specific IgG antibody concentrations measured by EIA are higher in symptomatic than in asymptomatic dairy herd workers.[8] Immunoblotting of serum from exposed farmers shows no major differences in reactivities between symptomatic and asymptomatic; all had antibodies to 11, 25 or 60 kd bands.[2,7] These commonly recognized antigens should be included in all preparations used for diagnostic purposes.[7] The negative predictive value of the absence of antibodies to all of these bands has not yet been carefully tested, nor has the negative predictive value of the absence of IgM RFs which are present in most patients with farmer's lung[2] or air conditioner pneumonitis.[9] IgM RFs in the presence of antigen-reactive IgG can sometimes give rise to false-positive IgM bands on immunoblots.[2] As yet, immunoblotting has no positive predictive value for HP; its negative predictive value using purified or cloned antigens is promising but unproven. DNA probe and PCR techniques are not yet developed. See in this Chapter: **Aspergillus spp.** and **Thermoactinomyces spp.**

REFERENCES

1. Kurup VP, Agre NS. Transfer of *Micropolyspora rectivirgula* to Faenia gen. nov. International Journal System Bacteriology 1983;33:663-5.

2. Aznar C, Andre PM, Deunff J, Robert R. Investigation of human immune response to *Micropolyspora faeni* antigens by enzyme-linked immunoelectrodiffusion assay and immunoblotting. J Clin Microbiol 1988;26:443-7.

3. Khan ZU, Gangwar M, Gaur SN, Randhawa HS. Thermophilic actinomycetes in cane sugar mills: an aeromicrobiologic and seroepidemiologic study. Antonie Van Leeuwenhoek 1995;67:339-44.

4. Gaur SN, Gangwar M, Khan ZU, Jain SK, Randhawa HS. Farmer's lung disease in north-western India—a preliminary report. Indian J Chest Dis Allied Sci 1992;34:49-56.

5. Kurup VP. Detection of relevant farmer's lung antigens by using immunoblots of two-dimensional electrophoresis. Diagn Clin Immunol 1987;5:25-9.
6. Denis M, Cormier Y, Tardif J, Ghadirian E, Laviolette M. Hypersensitivity pneumonitis: whole *Micropolyspora faeni* or antigens thereof stimulate the release of proinflammatory cytokines from macrophages. Am J Respir Cell Mol Biol 1991;5:198-203.
7. Iranitalab M, Jarolim E, Rumpold H, et al. Characterization of *Micropolyspora faeni* antigens by human antibodies and immunoblot analysis. Allergy 1989;44:314-21.
8. Gangwar M, Khan ZU, Gaur SN, Randhawa HS. Occurrence and significance of precipitating antibodies against thermophilic actinomycetes in the sera of dairy herd workers, Nangali, Delhi. Antonie van Leeuwenhoek 1991;59:167-75.
9. Banaszak EF, Thiede WH, Fink JN. Hypersensitivity pneumonitis due to contamination of an air conditioner. N Engl J Med 1970;283:271-6.

Hypersensitivity Pneumonitis

Claire H. Hashimoto, M.D.

Hypersensitivity pneumonitis (HP) is an immunologically mediated lung disease caused by exposure to inhaled antigen, including bacteria, fungi, animal protein, and insect proteins. Acute and chronic forms exit. The acute form usually presents with dyspnea shortly after exposure to the inciting antigen. The chronic form has a nonspecific presentation, and can be difficult to diagnose since there are no strict criteria for the diagnosis. There are a variety of respiratory conditions associated with exposure to environmental antigens. These include farmer's lung disease (FLD), pigeon breeder's lung disease (PBLD), HP due to fungal antigens, which include those causing woodworker's lung disease and those associated with humidity/water (hot tub lung disease, humidifier lung, and shower curtain disease).

Many antigens are known to cause HP. The most common is the antigen form moldy hay, *Faeni rectivirgula* (previously known as *Micropolyspora faeni*), which causes farmer's lung disease (FLD). *F. rectivirgula*-reactive antibodies to IgG, IgM, IgA and IgE classes have been found in both symptomatic individuals with HP and unaffected subjects.[1,2] There is non-compelling evidence, however, that the levels are higher in the symptomatic patients with HP.[3] Immunoblotting of serum (for antibodies to 11, 25, or 60 kd bands) reveals no major differences in reactivities between symptomatic individuals with HP.[1,2] These antigens should therefore be included in preparations used for diagnostic purposes.[1] Smokers with FLD have a more insidious and chronic presentation versus nonsmokers with FLD. In addition, the 10 year survival rates for smokers with FLD is 70.7% versus 91.5% in nonsmokers with FLD.[4] In addition to *F. rectivirgula*, *T. viridis* and *Aspergillus fumigatus* are noted as antigenic causes for FLD. *T. candidus*, *T. sacchari* (also a cause of moldy sugar can HP), and *T. viridis* are other thermophilic *Actinomycetes* bacteria which are important in HP. *Saccharomonospora viridis,* although not commonly associated with FLD, can cause HP, and occasionally, patients with FLD have antibodies only to these species.[5]

Proteins from pigeon droppings can lead to breeder's lung disease (PBLD). Precipitating antibodies to avian antigens are noted in 40% of individuals exposed to birds.[6] This finding, however, does not always imply disease. Absence of the precipitating antigen is helpful in excluding the diagnosis.[6]

Fungal allergens are know to cause HP. *Alternaria* spp. can cause woodworker's lung disease as well as IgE-mediated allergic disease which is common in individuals with atopic disease.[5] As mentioned above, *Aspergillus* include malt worker's (*A. fumigatus, A. clavatus*), tobacco worker's and compost lung diseases. *Cryptostroma corticale* from moldy maple bark causes maple bark stripper's diseases.[5]

Cladosporium spp. cause an HP known as hot tub lung disease as well as IgE-mediated allergic disease.[5] Types of HP caused by *Penicillium* spp. include cheese worker's, humidifier

47

lung, woodman's and cork worker's diseases. *Phoma* spp. cause an HP known as shower curtain disease.[5]

In acute HP, the onset of fever, dry cough, dyspnea and malaise occurs 4-6 hours after substantial exposure to the offending antigen. Chest X-rays reveal a diffuse finely granular infiltration. Chronic HP could be difficult to diagnose due to nonspecific presentation and lack of defined criteria in arriving at its diagnosis. Indolent onset of dyspnea and cor pulmonale may be presenting symptoms.[7] Precipitating serum IgG antibodies to the offending agent are usually present, which, together with the history of exposure, are important in arriving at the diagnosis.[8] The presence of precipitating antibodies by themselves are not diagnostic of HP, since many individuals who are sensitized to various agents never develop lung disease.[9,10] Absence of the precipitating antibodies with the presence of lung disease suggests a different disease process.

A broad spectrum of findings appear in HP ranging from a subtle to extensive picture. Histologic features include interstitial chronic inflammation, noncaseating granulomas, intraluminal budding fibrosis and interstitial fibrosis. The most prominent feature are often an interstitial and peribronchiolar infiltrate including lymphocytes, plasma cells, and macrophages. Eosinophils are uncommon. Poorly formed noncaseating granulomas are seen in two-thirds of the cases. In 60% of these cases, intraluminal budding fibrosis is noted and can result in bronchiolitis obliterans. Some cases with repeated bouts of HP progress to honeycomb lung with devastating pulmonary impairment.[7,11]

The histologic differential diagnosis include LIP, sarcoidosis, infection (AFB, *Pneumocystis carinii*, fungi), bronchiolitis obliterans with organizing pneumonia (BOOP), and usual interstitial pneumonitis (UIP). Collagen vascular diseases and drug reactions can have a similar histologic picture as HP.[7]

In summary, the key findings in arriving at a pathologic diagnosis are granulomas, intraluminal fibrosis, and history of antigen exposure. Laboratory evaluation for precipitating serum IgG antibodies to a panel of antigens known to cause HP is helpful in arriving at a diagnosis of HP. Cases of HP difficult to diagnose can require a more invasive procedure such as lung biopsy. Treatment involves avoiding exposure to the offending antigen. Steroid therapy can be administered to patients with acute HP and some individuals with chronic HP. In general, the prognosis is good and HP can respond well to steroid treatment. The best treatment is to identify and avoid the offending antigen.

REFERENCES

1. Iranitalab M, Jarolim E, Rumpold H, et al. Characterization of *Micropolyspora faeni* antigens by human antibodies and immunoblot analysis. Allergy 1989;44:314-21.
2. Aznar C, Andre PM, Deunff J, Rober T. Investigation of human immune response to *Micropolyspora faeni* antigens by enzyme-linked immunoelectrodiffusion assay and immunoblotting. J Clin Microbiol 1988;26:443-7.
3. Brummund W, Kurup VP, Resnick A, et al. Immunologic response to *Faenia rectivirgula* (*Micropolyspora faeni*) in a dairy farm family. J Allergy Clin Immunol 1988;82:190-5.
4. Ohtsuka Y, Munakata M, Tanimura K, et al. Smoking promotes insidious and chronic farmer's lung disease, and deteriorates the clinical outcome. Intern Med 1995;34:966-71.
5. Reyes HR. *Thermoactinomyces* spp. In: Peter JB, editor. Use and interpretation of tests in infectious diseases. Fourth Edition. Santa Monica: Specialty Laboratories, 1996:283-4.
6. Krasnick J, Meuwissen JH, Nakao MA, Yeldandi A, Paterson R. Hypersensitivity pneumonitis: problems in diagnosis. J Allergy Clin Immunol 1996;97:1027-30.
7. Fleming MV, Travis WD. Interstitial lung disease. In: Marchevsky AM, Koss MN, editors. Topics in pulmonary pathology. Philadelphia: Hanley and Belfus, Inc., 1996:1-21.
8. Salvaggio JE, Karr RM. Hypersensitivity pneumonitis: state of the art. Chest 1979;75:270-4.
9. Arnow PM, Fink JN, Schleuter DP, et al. Early detection of hypersensitivity pneumonitis in office workers. Am J Med 1978;64:236-42.

10. Fink J, Banaszak E, Baroriak J, et al. Interstitial lung diseases due to contamination of forced air systems. Ann Intern Med 1976;84:406-13.

11. Hargreave F, Hinson KP, Reid L, Simaon G, McCarthy DS. The radiological appearances of allergic alveolitis due to bird sensitivity (bird fancier's lung). Clin Radiol 1972;23:1-10.

Penicillium spp.

Herminio R. Reyes, Ph.D.

The most important class of aeroallergenic fungi is *Deuteromycetes* which includes *Alternaria, Cladosporium, Penicillium, Aspergillus* and *Phoma* spp.;[1] many of these fungi can induce hypersensitivity pneumonitis (HP).[2] Types of HP caused by *Penicillium* spp. are cheese worker's (*P. casei, P. roqueforti*), humidifier lung (*P. casei*), woodman's (*Penicillium* spp.) and cork worker's diseases (suberosis) (*P. frequentans*).[3-8]

Although EIA detects IgG antibodies and ID demonstrates precipitins to antigens of *P. roqueforti* and *P. casei* in serum and bronchoaveolar lavage fluid of individuals with cheese worker's and humidifier lung diseases,[6-8] the presence of antibodies is not diagnostic of HP, because these antibodies are naturally present in serum due to the ubiquitous nature of *Pencillium* spp. in the environment.[9] IFA titers $\geq$1:160 for *P. marneffei*-specific IgG in documented *P. marneffei* cases versus titers $\leq$1:40 in other persistent fever patients and healthy controls were reported; however, the test was evaluated in an area of low endemicity.[10] Major IgE-reactive 64 kd and 68 kd antigens of *P. notatum* identified by IB are found at comparable frequencies in atopic patients and blood donors.[11]

Corneal (*P. citrinum, P. expansum*) and systemic (*P. chrysogenum, P. spinulosum*) hyalohyphomycosis and mycosis due to *P. marneffei* are diagnosed by isolation, culture and histopathology.[12-17] Mycosis due to *P. marneffei* is rare and is reported only in individuals who live in or have traveled to SE Asia.[12,13] *P. marneffei*[12,18-27] and *P. decumbens*[28] infections are reported in HIV-seropositive and AIDS patients. See in this Chapter: *Alternaria* spp., *Aspergillus* spp., *Cladosporium* spp. and *Phoma* spp.

REFERENCES

1. Salvaggio J, Aukrust L. Mold-induced asthma. J Allergy Clin Immunol 1981;68:327-46.

2. Levy MB, Fink JN. Hypersensitivity pneumonitis. Ann Allergy 1985;54:167-72.

3. Dykewicz MS, Laufer P, Petterson R, et al. Woodman's disease: hypersensitivity pneumonitis from cutting live trees. J Allergy Clin Immunol 1988;81:455.

4. Schlueter DP. Cheese washer's disease: a new occupational hazard? Ann Intern Med 1973;78:606.

5. Avila R, Lacey J. The role of Penicillium frequentans in suberosis: respiratory disease in workers in the cork industry. Clin Allergy 1974;4:109.

6. Campbell JA, Kryda MJ, Treuhaft MW, Marx Jr JJ, Roberts RC. Cheese worker's hypersensitivity pneumonitis. Am Rev Respir Dis 1983;127:495-6.

7. De Weck AL, Gutersohn J, Butikofer E. La maladie des laveurs de fromage (Käsewascher-krankheit) une forme particuliere du syndrome du poumon du fermier. Schweiz Med Wochenschr 1969;99:872-6.

8. Solley GO, Hyatt RE. Hypersensitivity pneumonitis induced by *Penicillium* species. J Allergy Clin Immunol 1980;65:65-70.

9. Notermans S, Veeneman GH, van Zuylen CW, Hoogerhout P, van Boom JH. (1--5)-linked beta-D-galactofuranosides are immunodominant in extracellular polysacchardies of Penicillium and Aspergillus species. Mol Immunol 1988;25:975-9.

10. Yuen K-Y, Wong SS-Y, Tsang DN-C, Chau P-Y. Serodiagnosis of *Penicillium marneffei* infection. Lancet 1994;344:444-5.

11. Shen H-D, Choo K-B, Wang S-R, Lin W-L, Chang Z-N, Han S-H. Immunoblot analysis of components of *Penicillium notatum* recognized by human IgE antibodies. J Allergy Clin Immunol 1991;88:802-7.

12. Heath TC, Patel A, Fisher D, Bowden FJ, Currie B. Disseminated Penicllium marneffei: presenting illness of advanced HIV infection; a clinicopathologic review, illustrated by a case report. Pathology 1995:27:101-5.

13. Chan JKC, Tsang DNC, Wong DKK. *Penicillium marneffei* in bronchoalveolar lavage fluid. Acta Cytol 1989;33:523-6.

14. Gugnani HC, Gupta S, Talwar RS. Role of opportunistic fungi in ocular infections in Nigeria. Mycopathologia 1978;65:155-66.

15. Upshaw CB. *Penicillium endocarditis* of aortic valve prosthesis. J Thorac Cardiovasc Surg 1974;68:428-31.
16. Delore P, Coudert J, Lambert R, Fayalle J. Un cas de mycose bronchique avec localisations musculaires septicemiques. Presse Med 1955;63:1580-2.
17. Piérard GE, Arrese Estrada J, Piérard-Franchimont C, Thiry A, Stynen D. Immunohistochemical expression of galactomannan in the cytoplasm of phagocytic cells during invasive aspergillosis. Am J Clin Pathol 1991;96:373-6.
18. Hulshof CMJ, van Zanten RAA, Sluiters JF, et al. *Penicillium marneffei* infection in an AIDS patient. Eur J Clin Microbiol Infect Dis 1990;9:370.
19. Tsang DNC, Li PCK, Tsui MS, Lau YT, Ma KF, Yeoh EK. *Penicillium marneffei*: another pathogen to consider in patients infected with human immunodeficiency virus [Letter]. Rev Infect Dis 1991;13:766-7.
20. Remadi S, Lotfi C, Finci V, et al. Penicillium marneffei infection in patients infected with the human immunodeficiency virus. A report of two cases. Acta Cytol 1995;39:798-802.
21. Liu MT, Wong CK, Fung CP. Disseminated *Penicillium marneffei* infection with cutaneous lesions in an HIV-positive patient. Br J Dermatol 1994;131:280-3.
22. Supparatpinyo K, Khamwan C, Baosoung V, Nelson KE, Sirisanthana T. Disseminated *Penicillium marneffei* infection in southeast Asia. Lancet 1994;344:110-3.
23. Kok I, Veenstra J, Rietra PJ, et al. Disseminated *Penicillium marneffei* infection as an imported disease in HIV-1 infected patients. Description of two cases and a review of the literature. Neth J Med 1994;44:18-22.
24. Supparatpinyo K, Sirisanthana T. Disseminated *Penicillium marneffei* infection diagnosed on examination of a peripheral blood smear of a patient with human immunodeficiency virus infection. Clin Infect Dis 1994;18:246-7.
25. Sirisanthana V, Sirisanthana T. *Penicillium marneffei* infection in children infected with human immunodeficiency virus. Pediatr Infect Dis J 1993;12:1021-5.
26. Vartivarian SE, Anaissie EJ, Bodey GP. Emerging fungal pathogens in immunocompromised patients: classification, diagnosis, and management. Clin Infect Dis 1993;17:S487-S491.
27. Hilmarsdottir I, Meynard JL, Rogeaux O, et al. Disseminated Penicillium marneffei infection associated with human immunodeficiency virus: a report of two cases and a review of 35 published cases. J Acquir Immune Defic Syndr 1993;6:466-71.
28. Alvarez S. Systemic infection caused by *Penicillium decumbens* in a patient with acquired immunodeficiency syndrome [Letter]. J Infect Dis 1990;162:283.

Phoma spp.

Herminio R. Reyes, Ph.D.

The most important class of aeroallergenic fungi is *Deuteromycetes* which includes *Alternaria*, *Cladosporium*, *Penicillium*, *Aspergillus* and *Phoma* spp.;[1] many of these fungi can induce hypersensitivity pneumonitis (HP).[2] *Phoma* spp. cause HP known as shower curtain disease.[2] PCR amplification of fungal DNA is useful for typing isolates.[3] See in this Chapter: **Alternaria spp.**, **Aspergillus spp.**, **Cladosporium spp.**, **Penicillium spp.** and **Thermoactinomyces spp.**

REFERENCES
1. Salvaggio J, Aukrust L. Mold-induced asthma. J Allergy Clin Immunol 1981;68:327-46.
2. Levy MB, Fink JN. Hypersensitivity pneumonitis. Ann Allergy 1985;54:167-72.
3. Rollo F, Salvi R, Torchia P. Highly sensitive and fast detection of *Phoma tracheiphila* by polymerase chain reaction. Appl Microbiol Biotechnol 1990;32:572-6.

Thermoactinomyces spp.

Herminio R. Reyes, Ph.D.

Thermophilic actinomycetes, including *Thermoactinomyces vulgaris* and *Faenia rectivirgula* *(Micropolyspora faeni)*, are Gram-positive, endospore-forming bacteria,[1] which, together with *Aspergillus fumigatus*, are the most common causes of the hypersensitivity pneumonitis (HP) termed farmer's lung (FL).[2] In addition to *T. vulgaris* and *F. rectivirgula*, *T. candidus*, *T. sacchari*, *T. viridis* and *T. thalpophilus* are other thermophilic actinomycetes important in the pathogenesis of hypersensitivity pneumonitis.[3-5] Antibodies reactive with a 55 kd band are very common in sera from patients with FL,[3] but neither the positive nor negative predictive values are defined. Antibodies reactive with *T. vulgaris* and *F. rectivirgula* are predominantly of the IgG and IgA class in FL patients.[6] Antibodies to *T. sacchari* in symptomatic bagasse workers are more commonly detected by EIA (~82%) than by CIE (~60%), but levels are not higher in exposed, symptomatic than in exposed, asymptomatic individuals.[7] In contrast, *F. rectivirgula*-specific IgG antibody concentrations measured by EIA are higher in symptomatic than in asymptomatic dairy herd workers.[5]

F. rectivirgula, or antigens thereof, stimulate IL-1 production by human alveolar macrophages and high-level secretion of tumor necrosis factor-α from human alveolar macrophages and monocytes, implicating direct stimulation of cytokine release in the pathogenesis of HP.[8] The pathogenesis of HP is clearly complex; simple diagnostic tests related to humoral or cellular mechanisms are not yet available. More emphasis should be placed on the negative predictive values of antibody testing. DNA probe and PCR techniques have not yet been developed. See in this Chapter: *Aspergillus* **spp.** and *Faenia rectivirgula*.

REFERENCES
1. Goodfellow M. Actinomycetes systematics: present state and future prospects. In: Szabo G, Biro S, Goodfellow M, editors. Biological, biochemical and biomedical aspects of actinomycetes. Budapest: FEMS Symposium, 1986:487-96.
2. Pepys J, Jenkins PA. Farmer's lung. Thermophilic actinomycetes as a source of 'farmer's lung hay' antigen. Lancet 1963;2:607-11.
3. Ylönen JK, Ojanen TH, Jägerroos HJW, Mäntyjärvi RA. Comparative immunochemical analysis of five thermoactinomyces strains. Int Arch Allergy Appl Immunol 1989;90:405-10.
4. Husman K, Vohlonen I, Terho EO, Mäntyjärvi RA. Precipitins against microbes in mouldy hay in the sera of farmers with farmer's lung or chronic bronchitis and of healthy farmers. Eur J Respir Dis 1987;152(Suppl):122-7.
5. Gangwar M, Khan ZU, Gaur SN, Randhawa HS. Occurrence and significance of precipitating antibodies against thermophilic actinomycetes in the sera of dairy herd workers, Nangali, Delhi. Antonie van Leeuwenhoek 1991;59:167-75.
6. Ojanen T, Terho EO, Tukiainen H, Mäntyjärvi RA. Class-specific antibodies during follow up of patients with farmers lung. Eur Respir J 1990;3:257-60.
7. Boiron P, Drouhet E, Dupont B. Enzyme-linked immunosorbent-assay (ELISA) for IgG in bagasse workers' sera: comparison with counterimmunoelectrophoresis. Clin Allergy 1987;17:355-63.
8. Denis M, Cormier Y, Tardif J, Ghadirian E, Laviolette M. Hypersensitivity pneumonitis: whole *Micropolyspora faeni* or antigens thereof stimulate the release of proinflammatory cytokines from macrophages. Am J Respir Cell Mol Biol 1991;5:198-203.

Chapter 5
Other Allergic States and Sensitivities

Aspirin Sensensitivity Reactions

Herminio R. Reyes, Ph.D.

Aspirin (acetylsalicylic acid; ASA) produces a number of adverse physiologic reactions including aspirin sensitivity, which in the context of allergic disease and asthma, refers specifically to the induction of either urticaria and angioedema or rhinoconjunctivitis with bronchospasm.[1,2] Aspirin sensitivity is also referred to as a "pseudo-allergic reaction," because its pathogenetic mechanism is uncertain.[1] Proposed mechanisms include: cyclooxygenase blockade leading to an altered PGE_2 (bronchodilator) to PGF_2 (bronchoconstrictor) ratio; a shunting of arachidonate from the cycloxygenase to the 5-lipoxygenase pathway (a feature which is thought to be significant in light of the eosinophilia); and an unidentified viral infection in which altered prostaglandin regulation of cytotoxic lymphocytes is hypothesized.[1-3] The presence of mast cells (and increased tryptase) as well as eosinophils (and increased eosinophil cationic protein) in the nasal mucosa and periphery suggests a role of these cells in the pathophysiology of aspirin sensitivity.[1]

The clinical features of ASA-sensitive individuals include rhinitis due to vasomotor instability, nasal polyps, eosinophilia in nasal smears, abnormal sinus radiographs and a general association with chronic asthma.[1] ASA-sensitivity is associated with a number of NSAIDs including piroxicam, ibuprofen, indomethacin and imidazole salicylate, but not with hydrocortisone sodium succinate; high doses of acetaminophen (> 1000 mg) should also be avoided.[2,4-6] An oral challenge with aspirin followed by forced expiratory volume (FEV) measurements is the only definitive method for establishing ASA sensitivity.[3,7] Development of a definitive skin test and RAST are clearly indicated.[7] See Chapter 3: **Eosinophil Cationic Protein.**

REFERENCES
1. Kowalski ML, Grzegorczyk J, Wojciechowska B, Poniatowska M. Intranasal challenge with aspirin induces cell influx and activation of eosinophils and mast cells in nasal secretions of ASA-sensitive patients. Clin Exp Allergy 1996;26:807-14.
2. Stevenson DD. Aspirin sensitivity: respiratory and cutaneous manifestations. In: Middleton EE, Reed CE, Ellis EF, Adkinson NF, Yunginyer JW, editors. Allergy: principles and practice. Vol. 2. St Louis: CV Mosby, 1988:1537-54.
3. Dahlén B, Boréus LO, Anderson P, Andersson T, Zetterström O. Plasma acetylsalicylic acid and salicylic acid levels during aspirin provocation in aspirin-sensitive subjects. Allergy 1994;49:43-9.
4. Settipane RA, Schrank PJ, Simon RA, Mathison DA, Christiansen SC, Stevenson DD. Prevalence of cross-sensitivity with acetaminophen in aspirin-sensitive asthmatic subjects. J Allergy Clin Immunol 1995;96:480-5.
5. Feigenbaum BA, Stevenson DD, Simon RA. Hydrocortisone sodium succinate does not cross-react with aspirin in aspirin-sensitive pathients with asthma. J Allergy Clin Immunol 1995;96:545-8.
6. Senna GE, Andri G, Dama AR, Mezzelani P, Andri L. Tolerability of imidazole salicylate in aspirin-sensitive patients. Allergy Proc 1995;16:251-4.
7. Cîrstea M, Cîrje M, Suhaciu G. The diagnostic value of intradermal tests with penicilloyl-dextran and aspiryl-polylysine. Physiologie 1986;23:237-43.

Beta-Adrenergic Receptor Autoantibodies

Douglas C. Aziz, M.D., Ph.D.

The human heart contains both $\beta1$-adrenoreceptors and a significant number of $\beta2$-adrenoreceptors; both are mechanistically involved in the positive inotropic and chronotropic effects of beta-adrenergic agonists. A substantial proportion of patients with dilated cardiomyopathy have circulating autoantibodies against the $\beta1$-adrenoreceptor.[1] Methods used to detect these autoantibodies include ligand-binding inhibition, isoproterenol-sensitive adenylate cyclase activity, EIA with β-adrenoreceptor peptides and immunoblots.[2]

In chronic heart failure, the number of both $\beta1$- and $\beta2$-adrenoreceptors is reduced. $\beta1$-adrenoreceptors are decreased in all forms of heart failure; whereas, $\beta2$-adrenoreceptors are decreased in mitral valve disease, tetralogy of Fallot and end-stage ischemic cardiomyopathy.[3] β-adrenoreceptor autoantibodies are detectable in 30–40% of patients with dilated cardiomyopathy, ischemic cardiomyopathy (22%) and alcoholic cardiomyopathy (25%).[2,4]

Affected family members with familial idiopathic dilated cardiomyopathy have a very high seroprevalence of β-adrenoreceptor autoantibodies (62%) and unaffected members to a lesser extent (29%).[5,6] This higher-than-expected frequency in unaffected family members suggests that the autoantibodies can be detected before the syndrome is clinically manifest.

Patients with dilated cardiomyopathy have a higher frequency of HLA-DR4 antigen (40% versus 24% in normal subjects). Of the patients with HLA-DR4 and dilated cardiomyopathy, 60–80% have β-adrenoreceptor antibodies, in contrast to only 22–25% of HLA-DR4-negative patients.[7] Most of these HLA-DR4-negative patients with dilated cardiomyopathy are HLA-DR1. None of the patients with autoantibodies have HLA-DR3 antigen; whereas, 37% of patients who do not have autoantibodies have HLA-DR3.

An autoantibody that cross reacts with *Trypanosoma cruzi*, the causative organism in Chagas disease, is identified in about 30% of patients with Chagas disease;[8] both types of adrenoreceptor autoantibodies are detectable in chagasic patients.[9]

REFERENCES
1. Aziz DC. Beta-adrenergic receptor (and other hormone receptor) autoantibodies. In: Peter JB and Shoenfeld Y, editors. Autoantibodies. Amsterdam: Elsevier Science B.V., 1996:115-9.
2. Limas CJ, Limas C. HLA-DR antigen linkage of anti-β receptor antibodies in idiopathic dilated and ischaemic cardiomyopathy. Br Heart J 1992;67:402-5.
3. Brodde OE. Pathophysiology of the beta-adrenoceptor system in chronic heart failure: consequences for treatment with agonists, partial agonists or antagonists? Eur Heart J 1991;12(Suppl F):54-62.
4. Limas CJ, Goldenberg IF, Limas C. Autoantibodies against β-adrenoceptors in human idiopathic dilated cardiomyopathy. Circ Res 1989;64:97-103.
5. Graber HL, Unverferth DV, Baker PB, Ryan JM, Baba N, Wooley CF. Evolution of a hereditary cardiac conduction and muscle disorder: a study involving a family with six generations affected. Circulation 1986;74:21-35.
6. Limas CJ, Limas C. Immune-mediated modulation of β-adrenoceptor function in human dilated cardiomyopathy. Clin Immunol Immunopathol 1993;68:204-7.
7. Limas CJ, Limas C, Kubo SH, Olivari MT. Anti-beta-receptor antibodies in human dilated cardiomyopathy and correlation with HLA-DR antigens. Am J Cardiol 1990;65;483-7.
8. Bonfa E, Viana VST, Barreto ACP, Yoshinari NH, Cossermelli W. Autoantibodies in Chagas' disease. An antibody cross-reactive with human and *Trypanosoma cruzi* ribosomal proteins. J Immunol 1993;150:3917-23.
9. Milei J, Sánchez J, Storino R, Yu Z-X, Denduchis B, Ferrans VJ. Antibodies to laminin and immunohistochemical localization of laminin in chronic chagasic cardiomyopathy: a review. Mol Cell Biochem 1993;129:161-70.

Cellular and Humoral Metal Hypersensitivity

Emmanuel A. Ojo-Amaize, Ph.D.

There are numerous ways in which metal ions can interact with proteins.[1] Mercury (Hg) and gold (Au) form metal-protein complexes by binding with high affinity to thiol groups of cysteine.[1] Such metal-protein complexes can activate T cells either dependently or independently of antigen, or by superantigen stimulation.[1,2] The use of Hg and Au in medicinal preparations is well documented.[1] Hg is still being used as a preservative and as a form of dental amalgam. Hg compounds can induce contact sensitivity and glomerulonephritis in humans.[3] Au(I) salts are used as antirheumatic drugs and can cause adverse immune reactions such as contact dermatitis, stomatitis, pneumonitis, glomerulonephritis, increased levels of serum immunoglobulins, antinuclear autoantibodies, thrombocytopenia[1] and asthma in goldminers.[4] Renal tubular damage is reported in mice chronically treated with cadmium chloride ($CdCl_2$).[5] The mononuclear cell infiltrate involves the T cell-specific, $CdCl_2$-inducible stress protein Hsp70 on tubular cells.[5]

Occupational exposure to beryllium salts is associated with chronic interstitial, granulomatous lung disease. $CD4^+$ T cells from berylliosis patients react to beryllium salts in an MHC class II restricted manner.[6] There is a strong positive correlation between berylliosis and HLA-DPB1*0201 which carries a glutamate residue at position 69, but not with HLA-DPB1401 carrying a lysine at position 69.[7]

Silica (SiO_2), silicone (dimethyl polysiloxane), and sodium silicate (Na_2SiO_3) induce memory T lymphocytes of the $CD4^+$ phenotype in individuals with silicone breast implants.[8] Silicone hypersensitivity is associated with high levels of IL-1 and IL-1ra in circulation,[9] neurocognitive and neuroimmunological findings.[10] Silicone immune disease reaction, which is associated with production of autoantibodies to multiple endocrine organs, is compatible with an immune-mediated endocrinopathy.[11]

The frequency of metal allergy to nickel sulfate, potassium dichromate, cobalt chloride, palladium chloride and gold sodium thiosulfate is statistically significant in patients claiming various subjective symptoms related to dental restoration materials.[12]

Suppression of cell-mediated immune response as measured by cutaneous hypersensitivity reaction is reported in goats treated with lead and cadmium.[13]

Standard laboratory methods for the assessment of cellular and humoral metal hypersensitivity include EIA,[14] memory lymphocyte immunostimulation assay (MELISA)[15] and lymphocyte proliferation tests.[8,16]

REFERENCES
1. Griem P, Gleichmann E. Metal ion induced autoimmunity. Curr Opin Immunol 1995;7:831-8.
2. Schrallhammer-Benkler K, Ring J, Przbilla B, et al. Acute mercury intoxication with lichenoid drug eruption followed by mercury contact allergy and development of antinuclear antibodies. Acta Dermatol Venercol 1992;72:294-6.
3. Eneström S, Hultman P. Does amalgam affect the immune system. A controversial issue. Int Arch Allergy Immunol 1995;106:180-203.
4. Cowie RL, Mabena SK. Asthma in goldminers. S Afr Med J 1996;86:804-7.
5. Weiss RA, Madaio MP, Tomaszewski JE, Kelly CJ. T cells reactive to an inducible heat shock protein induce disease in toxin-induced interstitial nephritis. J Exp Med 1994;180:2239-50.
6. Newman LS. To be^{2+} or not to be^{2+}; immunogenetics and occupational exposure. Science 1993;262:197-8.
7. Richeldi L, Sorrentino R, Saltini C. HLA-DPB1 glutamate 69: a genetic marker of beryllium disease. Science 1993;262:242-4.
8. Ojo-Amaize EA, Conte V, Lin H, et al. Silicone-specific blood lymphocyte response in women with silicone breast implants. Clin Diagn Lab Immunol 1994;1:689-95.
9. Ojo-Amaize EA, Lawless OJ, Peter JB. Elevated concentrations of interleukin-1β and interleukin-1 receptor antagonist in plasma of women with silicone breast implants. Clin Diagn Lab Immunol 1996;3:257-9.
10. Brautbar N, Campbell A. Silicone toxicity as a result of silicone implants [Editorial]. Int J Occup Med Toxicol 1995;4:1-2.
11. Brautbar N, Campbell A. Silicone breast implant recipients and autoimmune endocrinopathy. Int J Occup Med Toxicol 1995;4:75-8.
12. Marcusson JA. Contact allergies to nickel sulfate, gold sodium thiosulfate and pallaium chloride in patients claiming side-effects from dental alloy components. Contact Dermatitis 1996;34:320-3.
13. Haneef SS, Swarup D, Kalicharan, Dwivedi SK. The effect of concurrent lead and cadmium exposure on the cell-mediated immune response in goats. Vet Hum Toxicol 1995;37:428-9.
14. Shen G-Q, Ojo-Amaize EA, Agopian MS, Peter JB. Silicate antibodies in women with silicone breast implants: development of an assay for detection of humoral immunity. Clin Diagn Lab Immunol 1996;3:162-6.

15. Stejskal VD, forsbeck M, Cederbrant KE, Asteman O. Mercury-specific lymphocytes: an indication of mercury allergy in man. J Clin Immunol 1996;16:31-40.
16. Ojo-Amaize EA, Agopian MS, Peter JB. A novel *in vitro* method for the identification of individuals at-risk for beryllium hypersensitivity. Clin Diagn Lab Immunol 1994;1:164-71.

Chronic Fatigue Syndrome

Linda D. Dearing, M.S.

The diagnosis of chronic fatigue syndrome (CFS) is currently based on the working definition developed and refined by the Centers for Disease Control and Prevention which describes fatigue of 6 months duration seriously interfering with the patient's life and without evidence of various organic or psychiatric illnesses that can produce chronic fatigue. Although there are numerous major and minor criteria associated with CFS, an important prerequisite is to rule out other potentially responsible conditions (e.g., multiple sclerosis, major depression or other neuropsychiatric syndromes, malignancy, endocrine disease, autoimmune disease, drug abuse or medication effects).[1-3]

The pathophysiology of CFS is unknown, but the nature of symptoms and its typical appearance following a viral, flu-like illness suggest a combination of infectious, immunologic and psychological factors. The infectious agents most commonly associated with CFS are Epstein-Barr virus (EBV), human herpesvirus-6 (HHV-6) and enteroviruses. Although, not generally considered imperative for diagnosis, the presence of antibodies to EBV early antigen in significant concentrations, might prove to be useful markers of the antiviral therapy.[5]

A highly sensitive and specific enzyme immunoassay demonstrated antibodies to HHV-6 early antigen are found more frequently in CFS patients (119/154 [77%]) than in controls (20/165 [1.2%]); a high percentage (93/154 [60%]) were positive for IgM antibodies to HHV-6 early antigen.[6] The recent evidence of brainstem hypoperfusion in all (67/67) of patients with CFS might reflect neuronal damage by a viral agent (especially herpesviruses such as EBV or HHV-6).[7]

Assays now available for viral mRNA, cell-free viral DNA and quantitative PCR indicate active HHV-6 infection.[8,9]

CFS is also associated with persistent enteroviral infection; serology for enteroviral VP1 antibodies was positive in 18/23 (78%) of CFS patients studied[10] and enteroviral product was detected by polymerase chain reaction in 36/88 (40%) of a chronic fatigue syndrome study group as compared with 3/126 (2%) of healthy individuals.[11] Controlled prospective studies of well defined patient groups are badly needed.

The relationship between CFS and immune dysfunction is still unclear. In one case study of 26 CFS patients, no significant differences in immune function were found between control and CFS patients, unless patients were subgrouped by type of disease onset (gradual or sudden).[12] Patients with sudden CFS onset had a cell surface marker and cytokine profile similar to that seen in acute infection. Other reports indicate that CFS patients manifest phenotypic, quantitative and functional abnormalities of natural killer cells.[13-15] Decreased CD8 suppressor cell populations and increased activation markers on CD8 cells suggest that immune activation may play a role in CFS.[15] There is recent evidence that humoral immunologic dysfunction could be involved in CFS as well. In a study of 60 CFS patients, autoantibodies to nuclear envelope antigens were reported in 52% (31/60) of cases.[16] The autoantibodies mainly targeted nuclear lamins, including nuclear lamin $\beta1$. It therefore appears that both cellular and humoral immunodysfunction are involved in CFS.

REFERENCES

1. Krilov LR. Chronic fatigue syndrome. Pediatr Ann 1995;24:290-4.
2. Fukuda K, Straus SE, Hickie I, et al. The chronic fatigue syndrome: a comprehensive approach to its definition and study. Ann Intern Med 1994;121:953-9.
3. Komaroff AL, Fagioli LR, Geiger AM, et al. An examination of the working case definition of chronic fatigue syndrome. Am J Med 1996;100:56-64.
4. Hellinger WC, Smith TF, Van Scoy RE, et al. Chronic fatigue syndrome and the diagnostic utility of antibody to Epstein-Barr virus early antigen. JAMA 1988;260;971-3.
5. Hermann Jr WJ. The Epstein-Barr virus and chronic fatigue syndrome [letter]. JAMA 1989;261:1277-8.
6. Patnaik M, Komaroff AL, Conley E, Ojo-Amaize EA, Peter JB. Prevalence of IgM antibodies to human herpesvirus 6 early antigen (p41/38) in patients with chronic fatigue syndrome. J Infect Dis 1995;172:1364-7.
7. Costa DC, Tannock C, Brostoff J. Brainstem perfusion is impaired in chronic fatigue syndrome. Q J Med 1995;88:767-73.
8. Knox KK, Harrington DP, Carrigan DR. Fulminant HHV-6 encephalitis in an HIV virus-infected infant. J Med Virol 1995; 45:288-92.
9. Secchiero P, Zella D, Crowley RW, Gallo RC, Lusso P. Quantitative PCR for HHV-6 and 7. J Clin Microbiol 1995; 33:2124-30.
10. PreedyVR, Smith DG, Salisbury JR, Peters TJ. Biochemical and muscle studies in patients with acute onset post-viral fatigue syndrome. J Clin Pathol 1993;46:722-6.
11. Clements GB, McGarry F, Nairn C, Galbraith DN. Detection of enterovirus-specific RNA in serum: The relationship to chronic fatigue. J Med Virol 1995;45:156-61.
12. Mawle AC, Nisenbaum R, Dobbins JG, et al. Immune responses associated with chronic fatigue syndrome: a case-control study. J Infect Dis 1997;175:136-41.
13. Caligiuri M, Murray C, Buchwald, et al. Phenotypic and functional deficiency of natural killer cells in patients with chronic fatigue syndrome. J Immunol 1987;139:3306-13.
14. Buchwald D, Komaroff AL. Review of laboratory findings for patients with chronic fatigue syndrome. Rev Infect Dis 1991;13:S12-S18.
15. Landay AL, Jessop C, Lennette ET, Levy JA. Chronic fatigue syndrome: Clinical condition associated with immune activation. Lancet 1991;338:707-12.
16. Konstantinov K, von Mikecz A, Buchwald D, Jones J, Gerace L, Tan EM. Autoantibodies to nuclear envelope antigens in chronic fatigue syndrome. J Clin Invest 1996;98:1888-96.

Contact Sensitivity

Emmanuel A. Ojo-Amaize, Ph.D.

A variety of cutaneous diseases resulting from topical exposure to foreign antigens or sequelae of skin infections are due to T-cell-mediated delayed-type hypersensitivity reactions. These include skin rashes due to contact sensitivity to chemicals, such as drugs,[1] metals (nickel),[2] cosmetics and environmental antigens. Vascular endothelial cells in the skin lesions produce cytokine-regulated surface molecules such as IL-2.[3] In allergic contact dermatitis lesions, IL-4 mRNA is most strongly expressed;[5] whereas, IFN-γ mRNA is the predominant cytokine in tuberculin reactions.[4] Overexpression of IL-10 mRNA in atopic dermatitis might contribute to the upregulation of humoral responses and the down-regulation of T_H1 responses.[4] Some allergic individuals have several types of autoantibodies, including IgE[5] and β-adrenergic receptor autoantibodies.[6] The importance of these autoantibodies in disease pathogenesis is yet to be proved. Laboratory methods for the measurement of cytokines include EIA,[3] quantitative PCR,[4] ^{3}H-thymidine incorporation (radioisotope-dependent proliferation) and flow cytometry.[1]

REFERENCES

1. Abdouh M, Krzystynak K, Flipo D, Therien HM, Fournier M. Cytometric profile or molebdenum-induced contact sensitization versus a strong allergen reaction to oxazolone in murine auricular lymph node (ALN) test. Int J Immunopharmacol 1995;17:545-4.
2. Kapsenberg ML, Wierenga EA, Stiekema FEM, et al. TH1 lymphokine production profiles of nickel-specific CD4+ T-lymphocyte clones from nickel contact allergic and non-allergic individuals. J Invest Dermatol 1992;98:59-63.
3. Hatao M, Hariya T, Katsumura Y, Kato S. A modification of the local lymph node assay for contact allergenicity proliferation assay. Toxicology 1995;98:15-22.

4. Ohmen JD, Hanifin JM, Nickoloff BJ,e t al. Overexpression of IL-10 in atopic dermatitis. Contrasting cytokine patterns with delayed-type hypersensitivity reaction. J Immunol 1995;154:1956-63.
5. Gruber BL, Baeza ML, Marchese MJ, et al. Prevalence and functional role of anti-IgE autoantibodies in urticarial syndromes. J Invest Dermatol 1988;90:213-7.
6. Kaliner M, Shelhamer JH, Davis PB, et al. Autonomic nervous sytem abnormalities and allergy. Ann Intern Med 1982;96:349-57.

Delayed-Type Hypersensitivity

Emmanuel A. Ojo-Amaize, Ph.D.

Considered the largest organ in the body, the skin is the primary barrier to the external environment. Cellular components of the cutaneous immune system include keratinocytes, epidermal Langerhans cells, intraepidermal lymphocytes, dermal lymphocytes and macrophages. The homing of some T cells to the epidermis can be controlled by specific adhesion molecules.[1,2] The major type of T-cell-mediated immune response in the skin is delayed-type hypersensitivity (DTH). DTH is a cell-mediated immune response that results from the activation of T cells and the secretion of cytokines. Activation of different subsets of T helper (T_H) cells leads to secretion of different types of cytokines.[3] Cytokines involved in a T_H1 $CD4^+$ cellular response profile include IFN-γ, IL-2, TNF-β, TNF-α, GM-CSF and IL-3. Cytokines involved in a T_H2 $CD4^+$ cellular response profile include IL-3, IL-4, IL-5, IL-6, IL-10, IL-13, TNF-α and GM-CSF. T_H2 type immediate IgE-mediated hypersensitivity immune responses are induced by aero-allergens such as animal danders, dust mites and pollens which underly the increasingly prevalent disorder, asthma.[3,4] Positive tuberculin reactions induce T_H1 type delayed-type hypersensitivity responses resulting in a T_H1 cytokine profile.[3] T_H1 immunity has the potential to inhibit atopic disorder by the repression of T_H2 immunity.[3]

The Langerhans-dendrite cell (L-DC) is a unique cell lineage distinct from the mononuclear phagocytes. L-DCs comprise the Langerhans cells of the skin (LCs), the dendritic cells (DCs) of the spleen and the "veiled cells" of afferent lymphatics. The LCs are seminal presenting cells (APCs) in presenting antigens introduced via the skin or other epithelia. They participate as APCs in the process of "peripheral sensitization" which involves the migration of T cells out of the blood into the dermis.[6] Upon exposure to contact allergens, but not to irritants or tolerogens, Langerhans cells show enhanced migration, possibly due to induction of IL-1β.[6] As a result of increased migration, paracortical T cells in the draining lymph nodes are activated and allergen-specific T-cell populations expand.[6]

DTH reactions peak at 2 to 3 days. DTH reactions are important for host defense against intracellular pathogens such as tubercle bacillus and are prevalent in certain diseases such as sarcoidosis and berylliosis,[5] Wegener granulomatosis and polymyositis.

The standard laboratory method for the detection of DTH is the lymphocyte stimulation test.

EFFECTS OF VARIOUS DRUGS ON IgE-MEDIATED SKIN TESTS[7]

Drugs	Suppression	Duration*
Anti-H_1 histamines		
Astemizole	4 +	5-40 days
Clemastine	3 +	1-10 days
Hydroxyzine	3 +	1-10 days
Chlorpheniramine	2 +	0.5 - 3 days
Promethazine	2 +	0.5 - 3 days
Tripelennamine	0-1 +	0.5 - 3 days
Diphenhydramine	0-1 +	0.5 - 3 days
Cyproheptadine	0-1 +	0.5 - 3 days

Drugs	Suppression	Duration*
Anti-H$_2$ histamines	0	
Cimetidine		
Rinitidine	2+	
H$_1$ + H$_2$ antihistamines	4+	> 5 days
Ketotifen	4+	>10 days
Imipramines	4+	
Phenothiazines	2+	
Corticosteroids		
Systemic, short term	0	
Systemic, long term	Possible	
Beclomethasone	0	
Theophylline	0-1+	
Cromolyn	0	
Beta$_2$ agonists		
Inhaled	0	
Oral, injection	0-2+	
Dopamine	1+	
Specific immunotherapy	1-3+	

*Duration of the suppression of skin tests varies among patients.

REFERENCES
1. Bevilacqua MP. Endothelial-leukocyte adhesion molecules. Annu Rev Immunol 1993;11:767-804.
2. Picker LJ, Butcher EC. Physiological and molecular mechanisms of lymphocyte homing. Annu Rev Immunol 1992;10:561-91.
3. Shirakawa T, Enomoto T, Shimazu S-I, Hopkin JM. The inverse association between tuberculin responses and atopic disorder. Science 1997;275:77-9.
4. Cookson WOCM, Moffatt MF. Asthma: an epidemic in the absence of infection. Science 1997;275:41-2.
5. Tinkle SS, Kittle LA, Shumacher BA, Newman LS. Beryllium induces IL-2 and IFN-γ in berylliosis. J Immunol 1997;158:518-25.
6. Bos JD. The skin as an organ of immunity. Clin Exp Immunol 1997;107(Suppl 1): 3-5.
7. Bousquet, J. In vivo methods for study of allergy: skin tests, techniques and interpretation. In: Middleton E, Reed CE, Ellis EF, Adkinson NF, Yunginger IW, editors. Allergy: principles and practice. St. Louis: CV Mosby, 1988:427.

Drug Allergy

Herminio R. Reyes, Ph.D.

Drug allergies, a diverse group of immunologic reactions with varied clinical presentations, are frequently associated with acute or chronic diseases.[1-3] Although the term "drug allergy" is common, reactions to drugs rarely involve Type I hypersensitivity; depending on the structure of the drug (small molecule, peptide or large protein), other immunologic reactions (type II-IV) are frequently encountered.[2] Major types of reactions studied in detail include those to penicillin, local anesthetics, insulin and vaccines as well as reactions to aspirin and sulfites.

For small molecules, possible mechanisms include haptenation (covalent linkage to other proteins), dehaptenation (reversal of attachment by plasma enzymes) and the production of reactive metabolic products through microsomal reactions. For large molecules, contaminants in commercial preparations can also confound *in vitro* analysis.[1-3] In drug allergy, in contrast to atopy, skin testing meets with variable success, being most useful with sensitivity to protein allergens such as insulin and chymopapain. RAST testing, which is available for various small molecules including beta-lactam antibiotics, sulfonamides, trimethoprim and isoniazid as well as several protein determinants, might not distinguish between major and minor epitopes of importance. A lymphocyte proliferation test, though impressive for some drugs,[3-5] is not widely useful. *In vitro* lymphocyte toxicity assays for hypersensitivity to anticonvulsants involve exposure of donor lymphocytes to microsomal metabolites of the drug, followed by assessment of lymphocyte toxicity.[6,7] Other tests of potential use are mast cell tryptase, C5a and C3a for assessment of anaphylactic reactions, assessment of classical and alternative pathways of complement activation for immune complex-associated reactions, measurement of prostaglandin D2 for mast cell activation, and assays for determining C1-C1 inhibitor and SC5b-9 membrane attack complexes.[1,2] See in this Chapter: **Aspirin Sensitivity Reactions** and **Penicillin Sensitivity.**

REFERENCES
1. Volz MA, Nelson HS. Drug allergy: best diagnostic and treatment approaches. Postgrad Med 1990;87:137-42, 149.
2. Sullivan TJ. Drug allergy. In: Middleton E, Reed CE, Ellis EF, Atkinson NF, Yunginger JW, editors. Allergy: principles and practice. Vol. 2. St. Louis: CV Mosby, 1988:1523-36.
3. Park BK, Coleman JW, Kitteringham NR. Drug disposition and drug hypersensitivity. Biochem Pharmacol 1987;36:581-90.
4. Zakrzewska JM, Ivanyi L. *In vitro* lymphocyte proliferation by carbamazepine, carbamazepine-10, 11-epoxide, and oxcarbazepine in the diagnosis of drug-induced hypersensitivity. J Allergy Clin Immunol 1988;82:110-5.
5. Houwerzijl J, De Gast GC, Nater JP, Esselink MT, Niewig HO. Lymphocyte-stimulation tests and patch tests in carbamazepine hypersensitivity. Clin Exp Immunol 1977;29:272-7.
6. Spielberg SP, Shear NH, Cannon M, Hutson NJ, Gunderson K. *In-vitro* assessment of a hypersensitivity syndrome associated with sorbinil. Ann Intern Med 1991;114:720-4.
7. Shear NH, Spielberg SP. Anticonvulsant hypersensitivity syndrome. *In vitro* assessment of risk. J Clin Invest 1988;82:1826-32.

Food Allergy

Herminio R. Reyes, Ph.D.

Although the majority of food-related allergies involve IgE-mediated (type I) hypersensitivity, type II (cytotoxic), type III (immune complex-mediated) and type IV (cell-mediated; delayed-type) hypersensitivity reactions to food allergens are noted.[1] Skin, gut and respiratory tract signs and symptoms are the most common, although other organs can be involved. A syndrome termed "exercise-induced anaphylaxis" characterized by erythema, urticaria, upper respiratory tract obstruction, and/or collapse in association with exercise is described; foods implicated include celery, shellfish, wheat, grapes, nuts, peach, egg, orange, apple, hazelnut, cheese and cabbage.[2]

Atopic sensitization to cow's milk is the most common food allergy;[3,4] casein is the major allergenic and antigenic protein in cow's milk.[3] Eggs, peanuts and cow's milk are responsible for ¯80% of IgE-mediated allergic reactions in American children; whereas, peanut, other nuts and seafood account for most reactions in American adults. RAST was reported to be 100% sensitive for diagnosis of milk and egg allergy in double-blind, placebo-controlled food challenged (DBPCFC) adults.[5] In other studies, RAST was not useful for diagnosis of food allergy in patients with rhinitis.[6]

DBPCFC is the gold standard for diagnosis of food allergy; however, the test is time-consuming, expensive and dosages/time intervals between challenges are not standardized.[4,7] In contrast to DBPCFC, RAST and allergen-specific IgE only measure type I IgE-mediated immediate hypersensitivity and anaphylactic reactions to food allergens.[4,7] Total IgE concentrations are neither sensitive nor specific for diagnosis of food allergy.[4]

Cross-reactions are reported between tomato fruit and grass pollen allergens,[8] carrot and grass/tree pollen allergens,[9] as well as between snails and house dust mite allergens.[10] Proteins with structural homology to latex are postulated to predispose to food allergy.[11] A report of elevations of fecal eosinophil cationic protein, tumor necrosis factor-α and α1-antitrypsin following food challenge in atopic eczema warrants further investigation.[12]

REFERENCES
1. Wyllie R. Cow's milk protein allergy and hypoallergenic formulas [Editorial]. Clin Pediatr 1996;35:497-500.
2. Caffarelli C, Terzi V, Perrone F, Cavagni G. Food related, exercise induced anaphylaxis. Arch Dis Child 1996;75:141-4.
3. Docena GH, Fernandez R, Chirdo FG, Fossati CA. Identification of casein as the major allergenic and antigenic protein of cow's milk. Allergy 1996;51:412-6.
4. Corey JP, Gungor A. In vitro testing for immunoglobulin E-mediated food allergies. Otolaryngol Head Neck Surg 1996;115:312-8.
5. Norgaard A, Bindslev-Jensen C. Egg and milk allergy in adults. Allergy 1992;47:503.
6. Trevino AJ, Rapaport S. Problems with in vitro diagnosis of food allergy. Ear Nose Throat J 1990;69:42-6.
7. Levy FS, Bircher AJ, Gebbers J-O. Adult onset of cow's milk protein allergy with small-intestinal mucosal IgE mast cells. Allergy 1996;51:417-20.
8. Petersen A, Vieths S, Aulepp H, Schlaak M, Becker W-M. Ubiquitous structures responsible for IgE cross-reactivity between tomato fruit and grass pollen allergens. J Allergy Clin Immunol 1996;98:805-15.
9. Gómez M, Curiel G, Mendez J, Rodriguez M, Moneo I. Hypersensitivity to carrot associated with specific IgE to grass and tree pollens. Allergy 1996;51:425-9.
10. van Ree R, Antonicelli L, Akkerdaas JH, et al. Asthma after consumption of snails in house-dust-mite-allergic patients: a case of IgE cross-reactivity. Allergy 1996;51:387-93.
11. Beezhold DH, Sussman GL, Liss GM, Chang N-S. Latex allergy can induce clinical reactions to specific foods. Clin Exp Allergy 1996;26:416-22.
12. Majamaa H, Miettinen A, Laine S, Isolauri E. Intestinal inflammation in children with atopic eczema: gaecal eosinophilic cationic protein and tumour necrosis factor-α as non-invasive indicators of food allergy. Clin Exp Allergy 1996;26:181-7.

Hyperimmunoglobulin E Recurrent Infection Syndrome

Herminio R. Reyes, Ph.D.

Hyperimmunoglobulin E recurrent infection (Job) syndrome (HIERIS) is a congenital disorder characterized by high serum IgE, chronic eczematoid dermatitis, recurrent skin and sinopulmonary infections and increased *Staphylococcus aureus*-specific IgE[1] as well as heterogeneous patterns of deficiency or non-deficiency of antibody-forming capacity.[2,3] Colon perforation,[4] acute respiratory distress syndrome due to methicillin-resistant *S. aureus* sepsis,[5] *Candida* endophthalmitis,[6] necrotizing fasciitis,[7] ventricular[8] and bronchial artery[9] aneurisms, fungal pulmonary abscess,[10] recurrent Staphylococcal peritonitis,[11] and peripheral blood mononuclear cell-mediated bone resorption[12] are also reported in HIERIS patients. IFN-γ, which is produced in normal amounts by mitogen stimulation of peripheral blood mononuclear cells (PBMC) in HIERIS, inhibits spontaneous production of IgE (as well as IgG1, 3 and 4) by B-cell preparations from patients with HIERIS who have high spontaneous production of IgE *in vitro*.[12,13] Although other cytokine might be involved, decreased IFN-γ secretion is believed responsible for the predominant T_H2 T-cells noted in HIERIS; IFN-γ decreases serum IgE in HIERIS.[12,13] See Chapter 1: **IgE and IgE Autoantibodies** and Chapter 3: **Phagocyte Disorders.**

REFERENCES
1. Leung DY, Geha RS. Clinical and immunologic aspects of the hyperimmunoglobulin E syndrome. Hematol Oncol Clin North Am 1988;2:81-100.
2. Sheerin KA, Buckley RH. Antibody responses to protein, polysaccharide, and ΦX174 antigens in the hyperimmunoglobulinemia E (hyper-IgE) syndrome. J Allergy Clin Immunol 1991;87:803-11.
3. Pherwani AV, Rodrigues C, Dasgupta A, Bavdekar MA, Rao ND. Hyperimmunoglobulin E syndrome. Indian Pediatr 1994;31:328-30.
4. Chen CM, Lai HS, Lin CL, Hsieh KS. Colon perforation in a patient with hyperimmunoglobulin E (Job's) syndrome. J Pediatr Surg 1995;30:1479-80.
5. Sato E, Yamamoto H, Honda T, et al. Acute respiratory distress syndrome due to methicillin-resistant Staphylococcus aureus sepsis in hyper-IgE syndrome. Eur Respir J 1996;9:386-8.
6. Haslett RS, Moriarty AP, Vijayadurai P, McGalliard JN, Chandna A. Candida enophthalmitis in Job syndrome [Letter]. Arch Ophthalmol 1996;114:617-8.

7. Misago N, Tanaka T, Takeuchi M, Oka S. Necrotizing fasciitis in association with hyperimmunoglobulin E syndrome. J Dermatol 1995;22:673-6.
8. el Noor IB, Venugopalan P, Johnston WJ, Froude JR. Ventricular aneurysm and myocarditis in a child with the hyperimmunoglobulin E syndrome. Eur Heart J 1995;16:714-5.
9. Connolly B, Manson D, Khattak S, Burrows P. Bronchial artery aneurysm in hyperimmunoglobulin E syndrome. Pediatr Radiol 1994;24:592-3.
10. Hall RA, Salhany KE, Lebel E, Bavaria JE, Kaiser LR. Fungal pulmonary abscess in an adult secondary to hyperimmunoglobulin E (Job's) syndrome. Ann Thorac Surg 1995;59:759-61.
11. Khan GA, Bank N. An adult patient with hyperimmunoglobulin E (Job's) syndrome, end-stage renal disease and repeated episodes of peritonitis. Clin Nephrol 1994;41:233-6.
12. Cohen-Solal M, Prieur AM, Prin L, et al. Cytokine-mediated bone resorption in patients with the hyperimmunoglobulin E syndrome. Clin Immunol Immunopathol 1995;76:75-81.
13. King CL, Gallin JI, Malech HL, Abramson SL, Nutman TB. Regulation of immunoglobulin production in hyperimmunoglobulin E recurrent-infection syndrome by interferon. Proc Natl Acad Sci USA 1989;86:10085-9.

Immunodeficiency Disorders

Madhumita Patnaik, M.D.

Immunodeficiency disorders are classified into four major categories based on recommendations from a committee of the World Health Organization. They are antibody (B cell) deficiency, cellular (T cell) deficiency, combined T cell and B cell deficiencies and phagocyte dysfunction.[1] Deficiency of one or more of these systems can be congenital,[2] or acquired. Immunodeficiency can be secondary to an embryologic abnormality, an enzymatic defect or can be due to an unknown cause.[3,4] The types of infections that occur and the physical findings are indicative of the type of immunodeficiency disease present. Several screening tests are available for each component of the immune system, which enable diagnosis in a great number of cases,[5] although there are others where the etiology is unknown. Therapy depends on the type of immunodeficiency and ranges from antimicrobial agents for the treatment of recurrent infections to immunotherapy, bone marrow transplantation, enzyme replacement and gene therapy.[6]

Classification of immunodeficiency disorders.

Antibody (B cell) immunodeficiency disorders
X-linked hypogammaglobulinemia (congenital hypogammaglobulinemia)
Transient hypogammaglobulinemia of infancy
Common, variable, unclassifiable immunodeficiency (acquired hypogammaglobulinemia)
Immunodeficiency with hyper-IgM
Neutropenia with hypogammaglobulinemia
Polysaccharide antigen unresponsiveness
Selective IgA deficiency
Selective IgM deficiency
Selective deficiency of IgG subclasses
Secondary B cell immunodeficiency associated with drugs, protein-losing sates
X-linked lymphoproliferative disease
Cellular (T cell) immunodeficiency disorders
Congenital thymic aplasia (DiGeorge's syndrome)
Chronic mucocutaneous candidiasis (with or without endocrinopathy)
T cell deficiency associated with purine nucleoside phosphorylase deficiency
T cell deficiency associated with absent membrane glycoprotein
T cell deficiency associated with absent class I or II MHC antigens or both (bare lymphocyte syndrome)
T cell receptor and signaling deficiencies
T cell deficiency associated with cytokine deficiencies

Combined antibody-mediated (B cell) and cell-mediated (T cell) immunodeficiency disorders
Severe combined immunodeficiency disease (autosomal recessive, X-linked, sporadic)
Cellular immunodeficiency with abnormal immunoglobulin synthesis (Nezelof's syndrome)
Immunodeficiency with ataxia-telangiectasia
Immunodeficiency with eczema and thrombocytopenia (Wiskott-Aldrich syndrome)
Immunodeficiency with thymoma
Immunodeficiency with short-limbed dwarfism
Immunodeficiency with adenosine deaminase deficiency
Immunodeficiency with nucleoside phosphorylase deficiency
Biotin-dependent multiple carboxylase deficiency
Graft-versus-host (GVH) disease
Acquired immunodeficiency syndrome (AIDS)
Phagocytic dysfunction
Chronic granulomatous disease
Glucose-6-phosphate dehydrogenase deficiency
Myeloperoxidase deficiency
Chédiak-Higashi syndrome
Job's syndrome
Tuftsin deficiency
Lazy leukocyte syndrome
Elevated IgE, defective chemotaxis, and recurrent infections
Immunodeficiency associated with natural killer cell defects

(Modified from Stites DP, et al. Basic & clinical immunology. CT: Apple & Lange, 1994:264.)

REFERENCES
1. World Health Organization Scientific Group. Primary immunodeficiency diseases. Immunodefic Rev 1992;3:83.
2. Featherstone C. The many faces of WAS protein. Science 1997;275:27-9.
3. Farrar JE, Rohere J, Conley ME. Neutropenia in X-linked agammaglobulinemia. Clin Immunol Immunopathol 1996;81:271-6.
4. Jaffe JS. T cell abnormalities in common variable immunodeficiency. Pediatr Res 1993;33(Suppl):S24.
5. Stiehm ER. New and old immunodeficiencies. Pediatr Res 1993;33(Suppl):S2.
6. Bordignon C, Notarangelo LD, Nobili N, et al. Gene therapy in peripheral blood lymphcoytes and bone marrow for ADA-immunodeficient patients. Science 1995;270:470-5.

Latex Allergy

Douglas C. Aziz, M.D., Ph.D.

Natural latex (NL), the milky sap from the rubber tree, *Hevea brasiliensis*, is a significant allergen, especially in health care workers. Symptoms range from hand dermatitis to life-threatening anaphylaxis. The prevalence of sensitized persons is about 3% in the general population, and 2% to 25% in various reports of health care workers. The prevalence of NL-specific IgE antibodies among nurses is ~9%.[1] Using a serum NL-specific IgE cut-off of ≥0.6 ng/mL, ~65% of health care workers have elevated concentrations.[2] Patients with frequent operations, such as children with spina bifida, have an increased prevalence of latex allergy (29%).[3] The number of operations and total serum IgE are the most important factors in predicting an allergy to latex.[3] NL-specific IgE is detectable by RAST, EIA, flow cytometry[4] and electrochemiluminescence;[5] the latter appears to have the greatest sensitivity.[5] Patients with latex allergy have increased frequency of allergy to foods, specifically avocado (53%), potato (40%), banana (38%), tomato (28%), chestnut (28%) and kiwi (17%), as demonstrated by skin prick testing.[6]

REFERENCES

1. Grzybowski M, Ownby DR, Peyser PA, Johnson CC, Schork MA. The prevalence of anti-latex IgE antibodies among registered nurses. J Allergy Clin Immunol 1996;98:535-44.
2. Kaczmarek DG, Silverman BG, Gross TP, et al. Prevalence of latex-specific IgE antibodies in hospital personnel. Ann Allergy Asthma Immunol 1996;76:51-6.
3. Nieto A, Estornell F, Mazon A, et al. Allergy to latex in spina bifida: a multireactive study of associated factors in 100 consecutive patients. J Allergy Clin Immunol 1996;98:501-7.
4. Sainte-Laudy J, Vallon C, Guerin JC. Diagnosis of latex allergy: comparison of histamine release and flow cytometric analysis of basophil activation. Inflamm Res 1996;45:S35-6.
5. Kobrynski L, Tanimune L, Pawlowski NA, Douglas SD, Campbell DE. A comparison of electrochemiluminescence and flow cytometry for the detection of natural latex-specific human immunoglobulin E. Clin Diagn Lab Immunol 1996;3:42-6.
6. Beezhold DH, Sussman GL, Liss GM, Chang N-S. Latex allergy can induce clinical reactions to specific foods. Clin Exp Allergy 1996;26:416-22.

Nasal Polyps Induced by Allergens

Claire H. Hashimoto, M.D.

Nasal polyposis is a chronic inflammatory disease of the paranasal sinus mucosa leading to the protrusion of benign edematous polyps from the meatus into the nasal cavities. These polyps are considered non-neoplastic and are hypertrophic swellings from an inflammatory process. Usually, nasal polyps can be diagnosed by nasal endoscopy. Nasal polyps are usually bilateral and grossly appear as smooth, pale, grapelike masses. If unilateral, biopsy is warranted to rule out a more ominous diagnosis, e.g., carcinoma.[1] Predisposing conditions for nasal polyps include cystic fibrosis (CF), asthma, and immune deficiencies.[2] In childhood, CF is the most common condition associated with nasal polyps. The severity of the disease wanes and increases with age, but nasal polyps develop early in these patients. One-third of adults with nasal polyps have asthma. Data indicate that IgE-mediated allergy seems to play only a minor role and does not explain the accumulation of eosinophils. Finally, individuals with immune deficiencies, both congenital and acquired, can have nasal polyps. These include those with primary ciliary dyskinesia and Young syndrome. Workup, including measurement of ciliary function and immunologic screening, is helpful in assessing these patients.[1]

Nasal polyps are covered with respiratory epithelium and are filled with edematous stroma and inflammatory cells. Eosinophils are characteristically noted. Nasal polyps can be categorized as edematous, cystic, or fibrous. A variable infiltrate of neutrophils, eosinophils, lymphocytes and plasma cells are seen. Eosinophils are more commonly observed in the edematous type of nasal polyp. The ciliated respiratory epithelium can have basal cell hyperplasia, squamous metaplasia, atrophy or ulceration. Occasional epithelial atypia can occur. Ducts are often observed and can be cystically dilated. The glands can show atrophic changes and occasionally hyperplasia. Stroma can contain fibrosis, especially when ulceration or infection has occurred. Rarely, the stroma contains large, bizarre, pleomorphic spindle-shaped cells with hyperchromatic nuclei and prominent nucleoli. Distinguishing this finding from a malignancy can be difficult. However, in the context of inflamed granulation tissue with infrequent mitotic figures, these cells represent bizarre reactive fibroblasts or histiocytes. Such findings in a nasal polyp do not indicate the lesion will recur or behave in a malignant manner.[3] Differential diagnosis of nasal polyps includes carcinoma, mesenchymal tumors (vascular, smooth muscle, skeletal muscle, fibrous tissue neoplasms), plamacytomas, malignant lymphomas and papillomas.

The etiology and pathogenesis of nasal polyps is unknown. There is a well-documented male predominance. Nasal polyps are not allergic in origin in the majority (two-thirds) of cases. Data indicates that IgE-mediated allergy seems to play only a minor role and does not explain the accumulation of eosinophils.[4] Many individuals with nasal polyps have a negative history of allergen-induced symptoms and negative skin and RAST tests, but have a significant number of eosinophils in their nasal secretions.[5] There is evidence suggesting that epithelial cells and fibroblasts from inflamed tissue can be upregulated *in vivo* and be the cause of inflammation in nasal polyps.[1] MG-CSF seems to play a central role. Studies show that GM-CSF mRNA can be detected in nasal polyps but not in normal nasal mucosa. About 30% of eosinophils in nasal polyps express the MG-CSF gene. Interestingly, epithelial cells do not show mRNA expression for GM-CSF; thus, eosinophils appear to play a key role. No difference between disease and normal tissue is found with respect to CD3, CD5, elastase-positive neutrophils and CD68-positive macrophages. There is evidence that IL-3 can play a role; the gene expression of this cytokine is correlated with activated eosinophils.[1]

Accumulation of eosinophils in nasal polyps is considered autocrine in nature. Eosinophils synthesize and secrete several inflammatory and regulatory cytokines including IL-3, IL-5, and GM-CSF. GM-CSF is stored within the crystalloid granules of eosinophils.[6] These three cytokines prolong eosinophil survival *in vitro* and enhance the metabolic and chemotactic functions. In this manner, a chronic, self-sustained, eosinophilic inflammation of nasal mucosa in maintained.

There is evidence that eosinophils can be important in the formation and growth of nasal polyps.[13] Activated eosinophils in the lamina propria of nasal polyps lead to an array of cytokines and basic granule-derived protein and lipid mediators. Transforming growth factor (TGF) can be involved in the chronic inflammation and fibrosis noted in nasal polyps. Approximately 50% of eosinophils in nasal polyps express the TGFb1 gene (detected by *in situ* hybridization and eosinophil cytochemical staining). Therefore, eosinophils can play a central role in inflammation plus matrix formation in nasal polyps.[3]

Potential mechanisms for selective eosinophilic accumulation in nonallergic nasal polyps include expression of vascular cell adhesion molecule-1 (VCAM-1) on vascular endothelium.[7] VCAM-1 mediates transendothelial migration of eosinophils and lymphocytes. VCAM-1 can be upregulated via several cytokines including IL-4, IL-13, IL-1β and TNF-α. A chemokine, RANTES, is elaborated within 24 hours of allergen challenge and is associated with influx of CD3$^+$, CD4$^+$, and CD8$^+$ cells locally and in the airways. There is evidence VCAM-1 and RANTES are important in nonallergic eosinophil infiltration. There is a strong association between TNF-α and the upregulation of VCAM-1.[7] Evidence for viral etiology as another possible mechanism for nasal polyp formation is noted in EBV studies. PCR analyses reveal 9 out 13 (69%) cases positive for EBV infection. *In situ* hybridization for EBV-encoded small nuclear RNAs (EBER) is positive in 11 of 13 (85%) cases of nasal polyps.[8] The virus is contained within a sparse number of stromal lymphocytes and not epithelial cells. Hence, the incidence of EBV positivity is high in nasal polyps (85%) with only very low numbers of EBV positive cells found in each case. This indicates that nasal mucosa could be a site of EBV persistence, thereby predisposing the region to developing viral associated tumors. It is known that EBV is strongly associated with nasopharyngeal carcinoma and nasal lymphoma. Of note is that EBV can be detected by PCR in 80% of normal nasopharyngeal tissue specimens from Chinese subjects without apparent EBV-related disease.[9,10] Thus, the etiology of nasal polyps with respect to EBV etiology remains obscure.[11] Analysis of 14 nasal polyps by PCR for *Mycoplasma pneumonaie* revealed positive results in 13 (93%) of the specimens and only 1 out of 7 (14%) control samples (obstructive turbinates).[11] This suggests the possibility that *M. pneumoniae* is involved in the etiology of nasal polyps. Because this study is small, further investigation is needed to substantiate this premise.

Although nasal polyps are considered non-neoplastic, clonal chromosomal changes can occur. There are case reports of multiple polysomies in children with nasal polyps. Karyotypic studies of nasal polyps in adults have also shown chromosomal abnormalities including polysomies and structural aberrations. The significance of the cytogenetic abnormalities is uncertain since the biologic significance of karyotypic changes in both neoplastic and non-neoplastic tissue is unknown. Multiple karyotypic changes are described in benign proliferations such as choroid plexus papillomas, thyroid hyperplasia and adenoma, and ependymoma. Furthermore, a study of normal kidney tissue showing trisomy 7 indicates that such karyotypic changes are not necessarily associated with malignancy. Nasal polyps can be another non-neoplastic condition associated with clonal numerical chromosome changes.[12]

It is difficult to predict recurrence of nasal polyps once they are surgically removed. Recurrence of nasal polyps is noted to occur between 1 to 51 years post-surgery with a median of 9 years. Severe recurrence is a problem in 5% of patients.[13] Conventional medical treatment includes corticosteroid nose drops for a month. Some nasal polyps resolve without treatment. Another corticosteroid regimen involves injections, followed by inhaled corticosteroid sprays for 1 year.[14] Similar results with respect to blockage are obtained with surgical removal.[15] Although claims that the sense of smell improved in the medication group versus the surgically treated group, the sensation was diminished over the course of 1 year. Patients with cystic fibrosis and nasal polyps who require surgery can be a distinct clinical subgroup within the spectrum of cystic fibrosis.[16] These patients tend to have better pulmonary function and nutritional status, however, they also have a higher degree of health care utilization, a higher rate of acute exacerbations, and a higher rate of *Pseudomonas aeruginosa* colonization. These patients are found to be frequently infected by two specific genotypes of *P. aeruginosa*: the Δ-F508/Δ-F508 and Δ-F508/G551D genotypes. These individuals are different from other CF patients in that the following clinical findings are observed in this group: lower sweat chloride levels, less severe symptoms of pulmonary disease, older age at diagnosis and overall improved survival.

REFERENCES
1. Jankowski R. Eosinophils in the pathophysiology of nasal polyposis. Acta Otolaryngol (Stockh) 1996;116:160-3.
2. Drake-Lee A. Magical numbers and the treatment of nasal polyps [Editorial]. Clin Otolaryngol 1996;21:193-7.
3. Ohno I, Lea R, Flinders K, et al. Eosinophils in chronically inflamed human upper airway tissues express transforming growth factor beta 1 gene (TGFβ1). J Clin Invest 1992;89:1662-8.
4. Shatkin JS, Delsupehe KG, Thisted RA, Corey JP. Mucosal allergy in the absence of systemic allergy in nasal polyposis and rhinitis: a meta-analysis. Otolaryngol Head Neck Surg 1994;111:553-6.
5. Jankowski R, Coffinet L, Audouy H, Folinguet B. Leucocyte compartments in the nasal secretion medium. Rhinology 1997;in press.
6. Kayab B. Eosinophils and cytokines. In: Basomba A, Sastre J, editors. ECACI '95 Proceedings. Bologna: Monduzzi Editore, 1995:103-10.
7. Hamilos DL, Leung DY, Wood R, et al. Eosinophil infiltration in nonallergic chronic hyperplastic sinusitis with nasal polyps (CHS/NP) is associated with endothelial VCAM-1 upregulation and expression of TNF-α. Am J Respir Cell Mol Biol 1996;15:443-50.
8. Tao Q, Srivastava G, Dickens P, Ho FC. Detection of Epstein-Barr virus-infected mucosal lymphocytes in nasal polyps. Am J Pathol 1996;149:1111-8.
9. Cheung WWWY, Chan ACL, Loke SL, et al. Latent site of Epstein-Barr virus infection. Am J Clin Pathol 1993;100:502-6.
10. Tao Q, Srivastava G, Chan ACL, Chung LP, Loke SL, Ho FCS. Evidence for lytic infection of Epstein-Barr virus in mucosal lymphocytes instead of nasopharyngeal epithelial cells in normal individuals. J Med Virol 1995;45:71-7.
11. Gur PA, Chakraverty A, Callanan V, Gurr SJ. The detection of Mycoplasma pneumoniae in nasal polyps. Clin Otolaryngol 1996;21:269-73.
12. Speleman F, De Potter C, Van Roy N, Laureys G. Multiple polysomies in nasal polyps in children. Cancer Genet Cytogenet 1996;90:86-7.
13. Drake-Lee A, Lowe D, Swanston A, Grace A. Clinical profile and recurrence of nasal polyps. J Laryngol Otol 1984;98:783-93.
14. Charlton R, Mackay I, Wilson R, Cole P. Double blind, placebo controlled trial of betamethasone nasal drops for nasal polyposis. Br Med J 1985;291:788.
15. Lindholdt T, Fogstrup J, Gammelgaard N, Komholm B, Ulsoe C. Surgical versus medical treatment of nasal polyps. Acta Otolaryngol (Stockh) 1988;105:140-3.
16. Kingdom TT, Lee KC, FitzSimmons SC, Cropp GJ. Clinical characteristics and genotype analysis of patients with cystic fibrosis and nasal polyposis requiring surgery. Arch Otolaryngol Head Neck Surg 1996;122:1209-13.

Other Food and Drug Additives

Herminio R. Reyes, Ph.D.

Reactions to food (or drug) additives other than sulfites are frequently reported.[1] Urticaria and angioneurotic edema are the predominant symptoms.[2-3] Rigorous evaluation of reactivity to additives, however, is rarely attempted. Of the many additives utilized, reactivity to tartrazine is the most studied, but even in this case, the correlation with urticaria and asthma remains somewhat tenuous.[4-6] Part of the problem is attributable to the varied provocative test procedures and the lack of appropriate *in vitro* tests. Skin test-positive patients do not always show hypersensitivity reactions when oral challenges are performed.[3,7,8] An isolated report of an additive-induced leukocyte inhibitory factor remains to be confirmed.[9] Nevertheless, reactions to additives should be considered in patients with urticaria and as a confounding variable in drug allergy.[2,5] Dietary elimination and forced expiratory volume (FEV) measurements after challenge is the only definitive method for detecting food and drug additive intolerance in asthmatic patients.[10]

SWEETENERS IN DIFFERENT ANTIMICROBIALS*[11]

Sweeteners	Antimicrobials							Total
	Amo	Amp	P	C	E	S	O	
	(11)	(10)	(12)	(19)	(18)	(10)	(11)	
Mannitol	5	1	0	0	1	0	0	7
Lactose	0	0	0	1	2	1	3	7
Saccharin	5	4	11	0	1	4	5	30
Sorbitol	0	0	0	0	1	3	3	7
Sucrose	8	9	12	18	14	7	6	74
Unspecified	0	0	0	0	3	1	0	4
None	0	0	0	0	0	0	0	0

*Amo: Amoxicillin; Amp: Ampicillin; P: Penicillin; C: Cephalosporins; E: Erythromycin; S: Sulfonamides and their combinations; O: Others. Numbers of preparations for which data were collected are listed in parenthesis.

FLAVORINGS IN DIFFERENT ANTIMICROBIALS*[11]

Flavorings	Antimicrobials							Total
	Amo	Amp	P	C	E	S	O	
	(11)	(10)	(12)	(19)	(18)	(10)	(11)	
Cherry	3	2	3	1	4	3	2	17
Wild cherry	0	2	0	1	0	1	0	4
Imitation cherry	0	0	0	0	0	2	0	2
Cherry berry	0	0	0	3	0	1	0	7
Banana	2	0	0	2	0	0	0	4
Strawberry	1	0	2	1	0	0	0	4
Orange	1	0	0	2	1	0	0	4
Peppermint/ Mint	1	0	3	0	0	1	0	5
Raspberry	0	0	3	0	0	2	2	7
Grape	0	0	1	0	0	1	1	3
Guar gum	0	2	0	0	0	0	0	2
Black currant	0	0	2	0	0	0	0	2
Imitation guarana	0	0	0	2	0	0	0	2
Blood orange	0	0	1	1	0	0	0	2
Tutti fruity	0	0	0	1	0	0	1	2

Flavorings	Antimicrobials							
	Amo	Amp	P	C	E	S	O	Total
Unspecified	2	4	3	6	12	1	6	34
None	0	0	0	0	1	1	0	2

* **Amo**: Amoxicillin; **Amp**: Ampicillin; **P**: Penicillin; **C**: Cephalosporins; **E**: Erythromycin; **S**: Sulfonamides and their combinations; **O**: Other flavorings: 1 (0.9%) each: Am: Bubble gum, Lemon; P: Cinnamon, Rootbeer, Berry cream, Sealva orange, Curacao, Black currant; C: Mixed berry, Fruit punch; O: Apple. Numbers of preparations for each data were collected are listed in parenthesis.

DYES AND COLORING AGENTS IN DIFFEENT ANTIMICROBIALS*[11]

Dyes/ Coloring Agent	Antimicrobials							
	Amo	Amp	P	C	E	S	O	Total
	(11)	(10)	(12)	(19)	(18)	(10)	(11)	
Red no. 40	2	2	9	8	5	5	4	35
Red no. 3	5	6	2	3	4	0	1	21
Red no. 33	0	0	0	0	2	0	0	2
Red no. 28	0	0	0	0	0	0	1	1
Yellow no. 6	0	2	3	7	4	3	2	21
Yellow no. 10	1	0	0	1	1	0	2	5
Yellow no. 5	0	0	1	0	0	1	4	9
Blue no. 1	0	3	0	1	0	0	0	1
Alum lake	0	0	0	0	0	0	0	1
Titanium dioxide	0	1	0	0	0	1	0	1
Invertone	0	0	0	0	0	0	0	2
Brown shade "R" Color no. 5470	0	0	0	0	0	1	0	1
Gray Opatint OD-7502	0	0	0	0	0	0	1	1
Unspecified	1	1	0	0	3	1	1	7
None	2	0	0	1	2	2	0	7

* **Amo**: Amoxicillin; **Amp**: Ampicillin; **P**: Penicillin; **C**: Cephalosporins; **E**: Erythromycin; **S**: Sulfonamides and their combinations; **O**: Others. Numbers of preparations for each data were collected are listed in parenthesis.

REFERENCES
1. Hannuksela M, Haahtela T. Hypersensitivity reactions to food additives. Allergy 1987;42:561-75.
2. Juhlin L. Additives and chronic urticaria. Ann Allergy 1987;59:119-23.
3. Bahna SL. Food sensitivity. Handling reactions to food and food additives. Postgrad Med 1987;82:195-9, 202-4, 209.
4. Moneret-Vautrin DA. Food antigens and additives. J Allergy Clin Immunol 1986;78:1039-46.
5. Simon RA. Adverse reactions to food additives. N Eng Reg Allergy Proc 1986;7:533-42.
6. Lowry MD, Hudson CF, Callen JP. Leukocytoclastic vasculitis caused by drug additives. J Am Acad Dermatol 1994;30:854-5.
7. Malanin G, Kalimo K. The results of skin testing with food additives and the effect of an elimination diet in chronic and recurrent urticaria and recurrent angioedema. Clin Exp Allergy 1989;19:539-43.
8. Wilson N, Scott A. A double-blind assessment of additive intolerance in children using a 12 day challenge period at home. Clin Exp Allergy 1989;19:267-72.
9. Warrington RJ, Sauder PJ, McPhillips S. Cell-mediated immune responses to artificial food additives in chronic urticaria. Clin Allergy 1986;16:527-33.
10. Hodge L, Yan KY, Loblay RL. Assessment of food chemical intolerance in adult asthmatic subjects. Thorax 1996;51:805-9.
11. Kumar A, Weatherly MR, Beaman DC. Sweeteners, flavoring, and dyes in antibiotic preparations. Pediatrics 1991;87:352-60.

Penicillin Sensitivity

Herminio R. Reyes, Ph.D.

Sensitivity to penicillin arises from haptenation to proteins via amide or acyl groups (major determinant) or via disulfide groups (minor determinants).[1] The terms "major" and "minor determinants" refer to the frequency of these linkages to proteins and not to their allergic potential. Skin testing to the both the major determinant (using benzylpenicilloyl-polylysine) and to the minor determinant (penicillin G potassium, benzylpenicilloate sodium and benzylpenicloyl-N-propylamine) is recommended for detection of penicillin sensitivity.[2-4] RAST testing using major-determinant-linked moieties is ~99% specific but only ~80% sensitive in detecting penicillin allergy.[5]

True penicillin allergy is probably overdiagnosed by RAST.[5] The allergic response to penicillin (as detected by RAST) can decline over time in some individuals.[6] A comparative evaluation of the predictive values of skin testing and RAST (using both major and minor determinants), IgE concentrations and other tests is needed. Cross-reactivity between penicillins and cephalosporins is documented *in vivo* as well as in the laboratory.[7]

REFERENCES

1. Harle DG, Baldo BA. Identification of penicillin allergenic determinants that bind IgE antibodies in the sera of subjects with penicillin allergy. Mol Immunol 1990;27:1063-71.
2. Ressler C, Mendelson LM. Skin test for diagnosis of penicillin allergy -- current status. Ann Allergy 1987;59:167-70.
3. Prieto Lopez C, Gamboa PM, Zugazaga Prieto M, et al. Study of various immunological parameters in the diagnosis of allergy to penicillin G and its derivatives. Allergol Immunopathol (Madr) 1990;18:141-8.
4. Silviu-Dan F, McPhillips S, Warrington RJ. The frequency of skin test reactions to side-chain penicillin determinants. J Allergy Clin Immunol 1993;91:694-701.
5. Worrall GJ, Hull C, Briffett E. Radioallergosorbent testing for penicillin allergy in family practice. Can Med Assoc J 1994;150:37-41.
6. Holgate ST. Penicillin allergy: how to dioagnose and when to treat. Br Med J 1988;296:1213-4.
7. Sullivan TJ. Drug allergy. In: Middleton E, Reed CE, Ellis EF, Adkinson FN, Yunginger JW, editors. Allergy: principles and practice. Vol. 2. St. Louis: CV Mosby, 1988:1523-36.

Sulfite Sensitivity

Herminio R. Reyes, Ph.D.

Sulfites or sulfiting agents (sulfur dioxide, bisulfite salts and metabisulfite salts), which are widely used additives in foods, beverages and common medications, can induce reactions characterized by urticaria, angioedema, laryngeal edema, asthma and anaphylaxis.[1] Although more commonly observed in chronic asthma patients (5–10% of adult and 35–65% of children with severe asthma),[1] sulfite reactions are also recognized in atopic and some non-atopic individuals. Mechanisms proposed for sulfite sensitivity include hyperreactivity (to sulfur dioxide generated from sulfites) involving afferent cholinergic receptors in the tracheobronchial tree; IgE-mediated reactions in a small subset of patients; and sulfite oxidase deficiency.[1] In allergic sheep, metabisulfite-induced bronchial responses are blocked by a bradykinin β_2-receptor agonist, pointing to a role of the kinins in mediation of bronchoconstriction.[2] Medications which are partially effective for treatment of sulfite sensitivity include cromolyn (mast cell stabilization), atropine (blockade of cholinergic sensitivity), oxepin (inhibition of histamine-mediated reactivity), and cyanocobalamin (assisted sulfite oxidation in sulfite-oxidase deficient patients). Diagnosis of sulfite sensitivity rests largely on metabisulfite challenge for which a standardized protocol is available.[3] The pharmacology points to a complex etiology in which multiple mechanisms might operate simultaneously; differences in the response to challenges should be expected in the same patient at different disease baselines.[2]

REFERENCES

1. Peroni DG, Boner AL. Sulfite sensitivity. [Editorial]. Clin Exp Allergy 1995;25:680-1.
2. Mansour E, Ahmed A, Cortes A, et al. Mechanisms of metabisulfite-induced bronchoconstriction: evidence for bradykinin β_2-receptor stimulation. J Appl Physiol 1992;72:1831-7.
3. Guidelines for the diagnosis and management of asthma. National Heart, Lung and Blood Institute. National Asthma Education Program. Expert Panel Report. J Allergy Clin Immunol 1991;88:425-534.

Wiskott-Aldrich Syndrome

Ronald A. Blum, Ph.D.

Wiskott-Aldrich syndrome (WAS), a life-threatening, X-linked immunodeficiency, affects cells of several different hemopoietic lineages including B and T lymphocytes and platelets.[1-3] The disease is characterized by thrombocytopenia, recurrent infections, and eczema. WAS patients are also predisposed to malignancies.[4]

Mutations in the recently isolated gene encoding the WAS protein (WASP)[5,6] cause abnormal expression of several cell surface molecules on B and T lymphocytes in patients with WAS; indeed, impaired CD43 glycoprotein expression on lymphocytes is a typical hallmark of this disorder.[2]

Although the mechanism is unknown, WASP might be involved in lymphoid cell signaling[1,7-9] and cytoskeletal organization.[8,9] Among the potential mechanisms are interactions with GTPases, which control cell morphology and mitogenesis.[7,9,10] More specifically, WASP appears to be an effector of the GTPase CDC42Hs, modifying the connections between the enzyme and the actin cytoskeleton.[10]

Treatment has included intravenous immunolgobulin and antibiotic prophylaxis in combination with splenectomy.[11] Mortality, however, is high among children.[12] Determination of the genetic defect makes possible prenatal and postnatal diagnostic assays for the identification of suspected disease.[4]

REFERENCES

1. Cory Go, MacCarthy-Morrogh L, Banin S, et al. Evidence that the Wiskott-Aldrich syndrom protein may be involved in lymphoid cell signaling pathways. J Immunol 1996;157:3791-5.
2. Gerwin N, Friedrich C, Perez-Atayde A, Rosen FS, Gutierrez-Ramos JC. Multiple antigens are altered on T and B lymphocytes from peripheral blood and spleen of patients with Wiskott-Aldrich syndrome. Clin Exp Immunol 1996;106:208-17.
3. Rocca B, Bellacosa A, De Cristofaro R, et al. Wiskott-Aldrich syndrome: report of an autosomal dominant variant. Blood 1996;87:4538-43.
4. Sullivan KE. Genetic and clinical advances in Wiskott-Aldrich syndrome. Curr Opin Pediatr 1995;7:683-7.
5. Greer WL, Shehabeldin A, Schulman J, Junker A, Siminovitch KA. Identification of WASP mutations, mutation hotspots and genotype-phenotype disparities in 24 patients with the Wiskott-Aldrich syndrome. Hum Genet 1996;98:685-90.
6. Schwartz M, Bekassy A, Donner M, et al. Mutation spectrum in patients with Wiskott-Aldrich syndrome and X-linked thrombocytopenia: identification of twelve different mutations in the WASP gene. Thromb Haemost 1996;75:546-50.
7. Aspenstrom P, Lindberg U, Hall A. Two GTPases, Cdc42 and Rac, bind directly to a protein implicated in the immunodeficiency disorder Wiskott-Aldrich syndrome. Curr Biol 1996;6:70-5.
8. Banin S, Truong O, Katz DR, et al. Wiskott-Aldrich syndrome protein (WASp) is a binding partner for c-Src family protein-tyrosine kinases. Curr Biol 1996;6:981-8.
9. Kolluri R, Tolias KF, Carpenter CL, Rosen FS, Kirchhausen T. Direct interaction of the Wiskott-Aldrich syndrome protein with the GTPase Cdc42. Proc Natl Acad of Sci USA 1996;93:5615-8.
10. Symons M, Derry JM, Karlak B, et al. Wiskott-Aldrich syndrome protein, a novel effector for the GTPase CDC42Hs, is implicated in actin polymerization. Cell 1996;84:723-34.
11. Litzman J, Jones A, Hann I, et al. Intravenous immunoglobulin, splenectomy, and antibiotic prophylaxis in Wiskott-Aldrich syndrome. Arch Dis Child 1996;75:436-9.
12. Wengler GS, Notarangelo LD, Berardelli S, et al. High prevalence of nonsense, frame shift, and splice-site mutations in 16 patients with full-blown Wiskott-Aldrich syndrome. Blood 1995;86:3648-54.

Chapter 6
Evaluation of
Inflammation

Acute-Phase Proteins

Alaa E. Ahmed, Ph.D.

Acute-phase reactants are released into the circulation after tissue injury or infection in a wide variety of acute and chronic diseases including cancer. Most members of the pentaxin family of acute-phase proteins (APP) are produced in the liver under the direct control of IL-6 (hepatocyte-stimulating factor).[1] IL-1 and TNF are potent stimulators of IL-6, the major mediator of the acute-phase response.[1] During acute-phase responses, IL-1, TNF and IL-6 are produced by monocytes; cytokine production, the number of monocytes and the differentiation of macrophages are well correlated. Serum IL-6 concentrations correlate with C-reactive protein (CRP) and other APP concentrations.[2] The APP family includes CRP, serum amyloid A (SAA) and prealbumin (transthyretin) which increase several 100-fold; ceruloplasmin, C3, and C4 which increase 50% or more; α1-acid glycoprotein, α1-antitrypsin, α1-antichymotrypsin, β2-microglobulin, retinol binding protein, transferin, haptoglobulin, albumin and fibrinogen (the major determinant of viscosity) which increase two- to fourfold. Despite a clear age effect on ESR, no such effect is observed on plasma viscosity, CRP or α1-acid glycoprotein.[3] The validity of CRP measurements as an objective index of inflammation (particularly in rheumatoid arthritis) was demonstrated in several studies; however, CRP synthesis and the acute-phase response in general are non-specific and can be interpreted in the light of full clinical information.[4] ESR, an indirect index of the APP concentrations, correlates most closely with fibrinogen concentrations.[5] APP in pediatric patients are important in diagnosing and following up the course of systemic infections. Lower values in preterm neonates than in term neonates are well documented.[6] Gestational age significantly affects the serum APP concentrations at birth and also at 3 months of age; adult APP reference ranges are not suitable for infants.

APP can be sensitive tumor markers; the α1-acid glycoprotein ratio: prealbumin ratio is higher in head and neck cancer patients than in controls. When the ratio is >6, there is a 25% survival rate at 2 years compared to 57% survival in patients with a ratio <6. CRP concentrations are used to classify gastric, colon and other gastrointestinal tumors; however, CEA is still the marker of choice for monitoring colorectal cancer.[7]

REFERENCES
1. Duff GW. Cytokines and acute-phase proteins in rheumatoid arthritis. Scand J Rheumatol 1994;23(Suppl 100):9-19.
2. Housssiau FA, Devogelaer JP, van Damme J, de Deux-Chaisnes CN, van Snick J. Interleukin-6 in synovial fluid and serum of patients with rheumatoid arthritis and other inflammatory arthritidis. Arthritis Rheum 1988;31:784-8.
3. Caswell M, Pike LA, Bull BS, Stuart J. Effect of patient age on tests for the acute-phase response. Arch Pathol Lab Med 1993;117:906-10.
4. Pepys MB. Rheumatoid arthritis: the role of acute-phase proteins. Br J Rheumatol 1993;32:S1-2.
5. Barland P, Lipstein E. Selection and use of laboratory tests in the rheumatic diseases. Am J Med 1996;100:S16-23.
6. Kanakoudi F, Drossou V, Tzimouli V, et al. Serum concentrations of 10 acute-phase proteins in healthy term and preterm infants from birth to age 6 months. Clin Chem 1995;41:605-8.
7. Schwartz MK. Acute-phase reactants as tumor markers [Editorial]. Cancer Invest 1995;13:444-5.

C3a, C4a and C5a Anaphylatoxins

Alaa E. Ahmed, Ph.D.

The anaphylatoxins C3a, C4a and C5a, bioactive fragments of the complement components C3, C4 and C5, respectively (which have a spasmogenic effect on smooth muscles), play a key role in mediation of immunologically provoked inflammatory responses.[1,2] The biologic functions, mediated through binding to specific receptors (C3aR for C3a and C4a; C5aR for C5a), involve phagocytic cell chemotaxis and activation, stimulation of lymphokine and cytokine release, and other cell activation events.[3] C4a production results from classical pathway activation; whereas, C3a and C5a are produced by activation of the terminal sequence through the classical pathway and/or the alternative pathway.[4] C3a, C4a and C5a are inactivated *in vivo* to the less potent forms C4a desArg, C3a desArg and C5a desArg by serum carboxypeptidase N cleavage of the N-terminal arginine.[3,4] C5a is rapidly cleared from the circulation by binding to neutrophil C5aR even before carboxypeptidase N inactivation,[4] is unlikely to be a clinically useful analyte.[4] C4a concentrations should probably not be used as a marker of classical pathway activation when there is confirmed or suspected renal disease because C4a is cleared by the kidneys.[4,5] In general, monitoring of complement activation with C3a is preferred over C4a and C5a assays.[4] Accurate measurement of C3a and/or C3a desArg is confounded by *in vitro* generation of C3a when blood samples are collected in EDTA tubes. Addition of the synthetic protease inhibitor FUT-175 (nafamostat mesilate [Futhan®]) to EDTA in the collection tubes minimizes spurious *in vitro* complement activation.[4]

Elevated C3a concentrations are found in most patients with active SLE; C3a concentrations start to rise 1-2 months before SLE flares (e.g., nephritis, pericarditis and/or cutaneous vasculitis), and are also elevated in pregnant SLE patients.[4] C3a is elevated in 33% of patients with non- immune nephropathy (polycystic kidney, hydronephropathy).[4] Elevated C3a is also reported in patients with rheumatoid arthritis, multiple sclerosis, Guillian-Barré syndrome, diabetes, neonatal bacterial infection, sepsis, acute respiratory distress syndrome, thermal injury and following different forms of extracorporeal circulation such as hemodialysis and cardiopulmonary bypass.[4] See Chapter 7: **Complement Components, Complement Split Products** and Chapter 2: **Mannan-Binding Protein.**

REFERENCES
1. Muller Eberhad HJ. Complement: chemistry and pathways. In: Gallin JI, Goldstein IM, Synderman R, editors. Inflammation: basic principles and clinical correlates. New York: Raven Press, 1992:33-61.
2. Whaley K. The complement system. In: Whaley K, Loos M, Weiler J, editors. Complement in health and disease. Boston: Academic Publishers 1993:1-32.
3. Kohl J, Bitter-Suermann D. Anaphylatoxins. In: Whaley K, Loos M, Weiler J, editors. Complement in health and disease. United Kingdom: Kluwer 1993:299-324.
4. Ahmed AEE, Peter JB. Clinical utility of complement assessment. Clin Diagn Lab Immunol 1995;2:509-17.
5. Abou-Ragheb HHA, Williams AJ, Brown CB, Milford-Ward A. Plasma levels and mode of excretion of the anaphylatoxins C3a and C4a in renal disease. J Clin Lab Immunol 1991;35:113-9.

Chemokines

Vellalore N. Kakanaiah, Ph.D.

Chemokines, a group of molecules which function in the recruitment and activation of leukocytes and other cells at sites of inflammation, possess the properties of both chemoattractants and cytokines.[1] Chemokines are subdivided into two groups: α-chemokines (C-X-C chemokines) primarily activate neutrophils, while β-chemokines (C-C chemokines) generally activate monocytes, lymphocytes, basophils and eosinophils. [1,2]

Chemokine receptors, their ligands and expression

Chemokine receptor	Ligands	Cellular expression
CCR-1	MIP-1α, MIP-1β, MCP-3, RANTES	Monocyte, T-cell
CCR-2A , B (MCP-1Ra,b)*	MCP-1, MCP-3, MCP-4	Monocyte, T-cell, Basophil
CCR-3 (CKR-3)	Eotaxin, RANTES, MCP-2, -3, -4	Eosinophil, Basophil
CCR-4	MIP-1α, RANTES, MCP-1	Basophil, T-cell
CCR-5 (CC CKR-5)	MIP-1α, RANTES, MIP-1β	Monocyte, T-cell
CXCR-1 (IL-8RA)	IL-8	Neutrophil, NK cell

Chemokine receptor	Ligands	Cellular expression
CXCR-2 (IL-8RB)	IL-8, MGSA, NAP-2, ENA-78, IP-10, Mig	Neutrophil, NK cell
CXCR-3	IP-10, Mig	Activated T-cell
CXCR-4 (Fusin, Lestr, humstr, LCR-1)	SDF-1	Widely expressed

MCP: monocyte chemotactic protein-1, -2, -3; **MGSA**: melanoma growth-stimulatory activity protein; **NAP-2**: neutrophil-activating protein-2; **ENA-78**: 78-amino acid epithelial cell-derived neutrophil activator; **IP-10**: interaction-inducible protein 10; **Mig**: monokine inducible by interferon (Modified from Mackay CR. J Exp Med 1996;184:799-802 and D'Souza MP, Harden VA. Nature Medicine 1996;2:1293.)
*old name

Blocking chemokine function can profoundly affect inflammatory responses. MIP-1α antibody treatment, for example, affects the recruitment of immune cells to a variety of inflammatory sites in mice.[3] IL-8 antibodies, in various animal models of ischemic reperfusion injury, inhibit neutrophil recruitment and decrease tissue damage.[3] MCP-1 antibodies inhibit delayed-type hypersensitivity-mediated inflammation in rats.[4] RANTES, MIP-1α and MIP-1β are soluble factors that suppress entry of primary strains of HIV-1.[5] SDF-1 is an extremely efficacious chemoattractant for T cells and plays a prominent role in B-cell development.[6] SDF-1 is a potent inhibitor of infection by lymphocyte-tropic HIV-1 strains.[7]

REFERENCES
1. Mackay CR. Chemokine receptors and T cell chemotaxis. J Exp Med 1996;184:799-802.
2. D'Souza MP, Harden VA. Chemokines and HIV-1 second receptors. Confluence of two fields generates optimism in AIDS research. Nature Medicine 1996;2:1293-300.
3. Strieter RM, Standiford TJ, Huffnagle GB, Colletti LM, Lukacs NW, Kunkel SL. "The good, the bad, and the ugly." The role of chemokines in models of human disease. J Immunol 1996;156:3583-6.
4. Rand ML, Warren JS, Newman W, Ringler DJ. Inhibition of T cell recruitment and cutaneous delayed-type hypersensitivity-induced inflammation with antibodies to monocyte chemoattractant protein-1. Am J Pathol 1995;148:855-64.
5. Cocchi F, DeVico AL, Garzino-Demo A, Arya SK, Gallo RC, Lusso P. Identification of RANTES, MIP-1 alpha, and MIP-1 beta as the major HIV-suppressive factors produced by CD8+ T cells. Science 1995;270:1811-5.
6. Bleul CC, Fuhlbrigge RC, Casanovas JM, Aiuti A, Springer T. A highly efficacious lymphocyte chemoattractant, stromal cell-derived factor 1 (SDF-1). J Exp Med 1996;184:1101-9.
7. Feng Y, Broder CC, Kennedy PE, Berger EA. HIV-1 entry cofactor: functional cDNA cloning of a seven-transmembrane, G protein-coupled receptor. Science 1996;272:872-7.

Cytokine Inhibitors

Emmanuel A. Ojo-Amaize, Ph.D.

Monocytes and macrophages produce prostaglandins (PGs), notably PGE$_2$, which might provide feedback inhibition of cytokine production *in vivo*. Inhibition of cytokine production is a potential mechanism by which PGE exerts its anti-inflammatory effects and may thus render orally active PGE analogs useful in the treatment of chronic inflammatory diseases.[1] Treatment of rats with a monoclonal antibody against murine IL-6, a major mediator of acute-phase responses, improves survival in *E. coli* shock.[2] Circulating adrenaline in septic shock might act as a feedback inhibitor of cytokine production. β-adrenergic agonists are reported to increase cAMP levels in THP-1 cells and to suppress production of TNF-α.[3] Inhibition of TNF-α production is abolished by a β-adrenergic antagonist, but not by an α-adrenergic antagonist; isoproterenol, a β-adrenergic agonist, inhibits TNF-α production. Dexamethasone and cAMP phosphodiesterase (PDE-IV) inhibitors (rolipram, nitoquasone) are reported to suppress the secretion of TNF-α by LPS-activated human monocytes.[4] The inhibitory effects of dexamethasone on the formation of IL-1α, IL-1β and IL-6 are also observed.[5]

Interleukin 1 receptor antagonist (IL-1ra) is the only recognized natural selective antagonist of a cytokine; its exclusive function is to block the binding of IL-1α and IL-1β to their cell surface receptors.[6] IL-1ra is under evaluation in clinical trials as a potential therapeutic modality in conditions characterized by elevated IL-1 production such as septic shock and rheumatoid arthritis.[7] Overproduction of IL-1ra is reported in 74% of women with silicone breast implants,[8] a condition in which silica and silicone are known to induce IL-1 generation.[9] Thus, the presence of IL-1ra in these women might have a beneficial effect by downregulating the adverse effects of IL-1β.

Antibiotics, such as fluroquinolones, clarithromycin and tetrandrine, inhibit production of IL-1 and TNF-α.[10] Besides antibiotics, opiate peptides (morphine) and antirheumatic drugs (gold, sodium thiomalate, auranofin) also inhibit TNF-α and IL-1β production by human peripheral blood monocytes.[11,12] Some of the anti-inflammatory drugs reported to have cytokine inhibitory capacities include 1X207,887, tenidap (a potent cox inhibitor which decreases levels of C-reactive protein via IL-6 inhibition), naphthalenylpropenoic acid derivatives and bicyclic imidazoles.[13] EIA is the gold standard for assaying cytokine inhibitors such as IL-1ra and IL-10.

There is a significant association between low concentrations of cytokine inhibitors in the lungs of patients with adult respiratory distress syndrome (ARDS) and subsequent patient mortality rate.[14]

REFERENCES

1. Goodwin JS. Are prostaglandins proinflammatory, antiinflammatory, both or neither? J Rheumatol 1991;28:26-9.
2. Starnes Jr HF, Pearce MK, Tewari JH, Yim JH, You JC, Abrams JS. Anti-IL-6 monoclonal antibodies protect against lethal *Escherichia coli* infection and lethal necrosis factor-I challenge in mice. J Immunol 1990;145:4185-91.
3. Severn A, Rapson NT, Hunter CA, Liew FY. Regulation of tumor necrosis factor production by adrenaline and beta-adrenergic agonists. J Immunol 1992;148:3441-5.
4. Molnar-Kimber KL, Yonno L, Heaship RJ, Weichman BM. Differential regulation of TNF-I and IL-1β production from endotoxin stimulated human monocytes by phosphodiesterase inhibitors. Mediat Inflamm 1992;1:411-7.
5. Amano Y, Lee SW, Allison AC. Inhibition by glucocorticoids of the formation of interleukin-1α, interleukin-1β and interleukin-6; mediation by decrease mRNA stability. Mol Pharmacol 1993;43:176-82.
6. Dinarello CA, Thompson RC. Blocking IL-1: interleukin 1 receptor antagonist in vivo and in vitro. Immunol Today 1991;12:11.
7. Ohlsson K, Bjork P, Bergenfeldt M, Hageman R, Thompson RC. Interleukin-1 receptor antagonist reduces mortality from endotoxin shock. Nature 1990;348:550-2.
8. Ojo-Amaize EA, Lawless OJ, Peter JB. Elevated concentrations of interleukin-1β and interleukin-1 receptor antagonist in plasma of women with silicone breast implants. Clin Diagn Lab Immunol 1996;3:257-9.
9. Miller KM, Anderson JM. Human monocyte/macrophage activation and interleukin-1 generation by biomedical polymers. J Biochem Mater Res 1988;22:713-31.
10. Roche Y, Fay M, Gougerot-Pocidalo MA. Effects of quinolones on interleukin-1 production *in vitro* by human monocytes. Immunopharmacology 1989;13:99-109.
11. Chao CC, Molitor TW, Close K, Hu S, Peterson PK. Morphine inhibits the release of tumor necrosis factor in human peripheral blood mononuclear cell cultures. Int J Immunopharmacol 1993;15:447-53.
12. Danis VA, Kulesz AJ, Nelson DS, Brooks PM. The effect of gold thiomalate and auranofin on lipopolysaccharide-induced interleukin-1 production by blood monocytes *in vitro*: variation in healthy subjects and patients with arthritis. Clin Exp Immunol 1990;79:335-49.
13. Lee JC, Badger AM, Griswold DE, et al. Bicyclic imidazoles as a novel class of cytokine biosynthesis inhibitors. Ann N Y Acad Sci 1993;696:149-70.
14. Donnelly SC, Strieter RM, Reid PT, et al. The association between mortality rates and decreased concentrations of interleukin-10 and interleukin-1 receptor antagonist in the lung fluids of patients with the adult respiratory distress syndrome. Ann Int Med 1996;125:191-6.

Heat Shock Protein Antibodies

Alaa E. Ahmed, Ph.D.

The heat shock proteins (hsps), also known as stress proteins, are among the most abundant proteins in nature. Hsps are also expressed by many pathogens[1] and are grouped into 4 families according to their molecular sizes: hsp90, hsp70, hsp60 and small hsp (<40 kd).[2] Mycobacterial hsp65 antibodies are reported in rheumatoid arthritis, atherosclerosis, multiple sclerosis, Alzheimer disease and Parkinson disease.[3] Human hsp antibodies are elevated in a wide variety of inflammatory, autoimmune and infectious diseases.[2] The method of choice for detection and quantitation of hsp antibodies is EIA using purified or recombinant antigens. No clinical utility or diagnostic value is reported for hsp antibodies due to the overlap in reactivity and concentrations between normal subjects and patients.[2]

REFERENCES
1. Hartel FU, Hlodan R, Langer T. Molecular chaperones in protein folding: the art of avoiding sticky situations. Trends Biochem Sci 1994;19:20-5.
2. Rowley MJ, Karopoulos C. Heat shock protein antibodies. In: Peter JB, Shoenfeld Y, editors. Autoantibodies. Amsterdam: Elsevier Science B.V., 1996:336-42.
3. Gao YL, Raine CS, Brosnan CF. Humoral response to hsp 65 in multiple sclerosis and other neurologic conditions. Neurology 1994;44:941-6.

Interleukin 1

Vellalore N. Kakanaiah, Ph.D.

Interleukin 1 (IL-1), an inflammatory cytokine comprised of two polypeptides, IL-1α and IL-1β,[1] which recognize the same cell surface receptor,[1] is produced by a variety of cells in response to infection, microbial toxins, inflammatory agents, products of activated lymphocytes, complement and clotting compounds.[1] Cells known to produce IL-1 include osteoblasts, monocytes, macrophages, PMN, keratinocytes, Kupffer cells, hepatocytes, thymic and salivary gland epithelium, fibroblasts and glial cells (Schwann cells, oligodendrocytes, astrocytes and microglia).[2-13] In addition to inflammatory responses, IL-1 production is also upregulated during bone formation, the menstrual cycle, and in response to nervous system stimulation.[2,14,15]

The local release of IL-1 during cutaneous allergic reactions probably contributes to IgE-dependent inflammation, and intrarenal production of IL-1 contributes to glomerular injury.[16,17] Plasma concentrations of IL-1β, which are increased in rheumatoid arthritis (RA), but not scleroderma[18] or chronic fatigue syndrome[19] correlate with disease activity.[20] Synovial fluid IL-1 concentration is increased in RA.[21] Serum IL-1 concentrations are increased during the acute phase of Kawasaki disease[22] and are increased (with TNF-α) in children with severe infectious purpura.[23] IL-1β and TNF are often increased in cerebrospinal fluid in bacterial meningitis.[24] Plasma IL-1 (EDTA/aprotinin) is probably more appropriate for study than serum.[25] Antibodies to IL-1α are reported in rheumatic disease, hemodialysis patients and in some normal sera.[26,27] Blockade of the IL-1 receptor is expected to be an important approach to the treatment of several diseases. Plasma concentrations of IL-1β but not IL-1α which is largely cell-associated for several hours after endotoxin administration, are elevated two-fold after endotoxin infusion and are three to fourfold elevated in septic shock, where higher concentrations are found in surviving patients.[28] Circulating IL-1 might contribute to weight loss in cancer.[29] Elevated plasma concentrations of IL-1β and IL-1ra are reported in symptomatic women with silicone breast implants.[30]

The biological effects of IL-1 vary from inducing specific cell type responses to targeting entire systems and acting as endogenous pyrogen and somnogen.[1] Inappropriate or prolonged production of IL-1 is implicated in the production of a variety of pathological conditions including sepsis, rheumatoid arthritis, inflammatory bowel disease, acute and chronic myelogenous leukemia, insulin-dependent diabetes mellitus and atherosclerosis.[31]

REFERENCES

1. Dinarello CA. Interleukin-1. Adv Pharmacol 1994;25:21-51.
2. Dodds RA, Merry K, Littlewood A, Gowen M. Expression of mRNA for IL1 beta, IL6 and TGF beta 1 in developing human bone and cartilage. J Histochem Cytochem 1994;42:733-44.
3. Mallardo M, Giordano V, Dragonetti E, Scala G, Quinto I. DNA damaging agents increase the stability of interleukin-1 alpha, interleukin-1 beta, and interleukin-6 transcripts and the production of the relative proteins. J Biol Chem 1994;269:14899-904.
4. Foss HD, Herbst H, Hummel M, et al. Patterns of cytokine gene expression in infectious mononucleosis. Blood 1994;83:707-12.
5. Fernandez MC, Walters J, Marucha P. Transcriptional and post-transcriptional regulation of GM-CSF-induced IL-1 beta gene expression in PMN. J Leukoc Biol 1996;59:598-603.
6. Kameda K, Sato K. Regulation of IL-1 alpha expression in human keratinocytes: transcriptional activation of the IL-1 gene by TNF-alpha, LPs, and IL-1 alpha. Lymphokine Cytokine Res 1994;13:29-35.
7. Takacs L, Kovacs EJ, Smith MR, Young HA, Durum SK. Detection of IL-1 alpha and IL-1 beta gene expression by in situ hybridization. Tissue localization of IL-1 mRNA in the normal C57BL/6 mouse. J Immunol 1988;141:3081-95.
8. Tsukui T, Kikuchi K, Mabuchi A, et al. Production of interleukin-1 by primary cultured parenchymal liver cells (hepatocytes). Exp Cell Res 1994;210:172-6.
9. Fernandez E, Vicente A, Zapata A, et al. Establishment and characterization of cloned human thymic epithelial cell lines. Analysis of adhesion molecule expression and cytokine production. Blood 1994;83:3245-54.
10. Fox RI, Kang HI, Ando D, Abrams J, Pisa E. Cytokine mRNA expression in salivary gland biopsies of Sjogren's syndrome. J Immunol 1994;152:5532-9.
11. Fini ME, Strissel KJ, Girard MT, Mays JW, Rinehart WB. Interleukin 1 alpha mediates collagenase synthesis stimulated by phorbol 12-myristate 13-acetate. J Biol Chem 1994;269:11291-8.
12. Bergsteinsdottir K, Kingston A, Mirsky R, Jessen KR. Rat Schwann cells produce interleukin-1. J Neuroimmunol 1991;34:15-23.
13. Da Cunha A, Jefferson JA, Jackson RW, Vitkovic L. Glial cell-specific mechanisms of TGF-beta 1 induction by IL-1 in cerebral cortex. J Neuroimmunol 1993;42:71-85.
14. Lynch EA, Dinarello CA, Cannon JG. Gender differences in IL-1 alpha, IL-1 beta, and IL-1 receptor antagonist secretion from mononuclear cells and urinary excretion. J Immunol 1994;153:300-6.
15. Lotz M, Vaughan JH, Carson DA. Effect of neuropeptides on production of inflammatory cytokines by human monocytes. Science 1988;241:1218-21.
16. Bochner BS, Charlesworth EN, Lichtenstein LM, et al. Interleukin-1 is released at sites of human cutaneous allergic reactions. J Allergy Clin Immunol 1990;86:830-9.
17. Sedor JR, Nakazato Y, Knieczkowski M. Interleukin-1 and the mesangial cell. Kidney Int 1992;41:595-9.
18. Needleman BW, Wigley FM, Stair RW. Interleukin-1, interleukin-2, interleukin-4, interleukin-6, tumor necrosis factor α, and interferon-γ levels in sera from patients with scleroderma. Arthritis Rheum 1992;35:67-72.
19. Linde A, Andersson B, Svenson SB, et al. Serum levels of lymphokines and soluble cellular receptors in primary Epstein-Barr virus infection and in patients with chronic fatigue syndrome. J Infect Dis 1992;165:994-1000.
20. Eastgate JA, Symons JA, Wood NC, Grinlinton FM, Di Giovine FS, Duff GW. Correlation of plasma interleukin 1 levels with disease activity in rheumatoid arthritis. Lancet 1988;2:706-9.
21. McNiff PA, Stewart C, Sullivan J, Showell HJ, Gabel CA. Synovial fluid from rheumatoid arthritis patients contains sufficient levels of IL-1 beta and IL-6 to promote production of serum amyloid A by HEp3B cells. Cytokine 1995;7:209-19.
22. Maury CPJ, Salo E, Pelkonen P. Circulating interleukin-1β in patients with Kawasaki disease [Letter]. N Engl J Med 1988;319:1670-1.
23. Girardin E, Grau GE, Dayer J-M, Roux-Lombard P, The J5 Study Group, Lambert P-H. Tumor necrosis factor and interleukin-1 in the serum of children with severe infectious purpura. N Engl J Med 1988;319:397-400.
24. Low PS, Lee BW, Yap KH, Tay, JS, et al. Inflammatory response in bacterial meningitis: cytokine levels in the cerebrospinal fluid. Ann Trop Paediatr 1995;15:55-9.
25. Cannon JG, van der Meer JWM, Kwiatkowski D, et al. Interleukin-1ß in human plasma: optimization of blood collection, plasma extraction, and radioimmunoassay methods. Lymphokine Res 1988;7:457-67.
26. Suzuki H, Ayabe T, Kamimura J, Kashiwagi H. Anti-IL-1α autoantibodies in patients with rheumatic diseases and in healthy subjects. Clin Exp Immunol 1991;85:407-12.
27. Sunder-Plassmann G, Sedlacek PL, Sunder-Plassmann R, et al. Anti-interleukin-1α autoantibodies in hemodialysis patients. Kidney Int 1991;40:787-91.

28. Cannon JG, Tompkins RG, Gelfand JA, et al. Circulating interleukin-1 and tumor necrosis factor in septic shock and experimental endotoxin fever. J Infect Dis 1990;161:79-84.
29. Belizario JE, Katz E, Chenker E, Raw I. Bioactivity of skeletal muscle proteolysis-inducing factors in the plasma proteins from cancer patients with weight loss. Br J Cancer 1991;63:705-10.
30. Ojo-Amaize EA, Lawless OA, Peter JB. Elevated concentrations of interleukin-1J and interleukin-1 receptor antagonist in plasma of women with silicone breast implants. Clin Diagn Lab Immunol 1996;3:257-9.
31. Dinarello CA. Role of interleukin-1 in infectious diseases. Immunol Rev 1992;127:119-46.

Interleukin 1 Receptor Antagonists

Vellalore N. Kakanaiah, Ph.D.

Interleukin 1 receptor antagonist (IL-1ra) is a naturally occurring receptor antagonist that binds IL-1R type I (IL-1RI) and, less avidly, IL-1RII without any antagonist activity.[1] Three isoforms of IL-1ra are known: a secretory form (SIL-1ra) which is produced and secreted by activated monocytes/macrophages;[2] an intracellular form (icIL-1raI), which is synthesized by epithelial cells;[3] and another intracellular form (icIL-1raII), which is produced by differential splicing in polymorphonuclear cells.[4] sIL-1ra inhibits the binding of IL-1 to its receptor, thus suppressing the biological activity of IL-1;[1] whereas, the actual biological significance of icIL-1ra remains unclear.[4]

A significantly higher serum concentration of IL-1ra is a pathophysiologic feature of active SLE and a good indicator of disease activity.[5] Similarly, synovial fluid from >80% of rheumatoid arthritis patients have elevated concentrations of IL-1ra compared with other arthropathies.[6] Elevated concentrations of both IL-1β and IL-1ra can be detected in plasma from women with silicone breast implants.[7] In adult respiratory distress syndrome (ARDS), concentrations of IL-1ra within the alveolar air spaces correlate with survival, suggesting that failure to mount a localized anti-inflammatory response early in the pathogenesis of established ARDS leads to a worse overall prognosis.[8]

REFERENCES
1. Arend WP. Interleukin-1 receptor antagonist. Adv Immun 1993;54:167-227.
2. Eisenberg SP, Evans RJ, Arend WP, et al. Primary structure and functional expression from complementary DNA of a human interleukin-1 receptor antagonist. Nature 1990;343:341-6.
3. Haskill S, Martin G, Van Le L, et al. cDNA cloning of an intracellular form of the human interleukin-1 receptor antagonist associated with epithelium. Proc Natl Acad Sci USA 1991;88:3681-5.
4. Muzio M, Polentarutti N, Sironi M, et al. Cloning and characterization of a new isoform of the interleukin 1 receptor antagonist. J Exp Med 1995;182:623-8.
5. Suzuki H, Takemura H, Kashiwagi H. Interleukin-1 receptor antagonist in patient with active systemic lupus erythematosus. Arthritis Rheum 1995;38:1055-9.
6. Malyak M, Swaney RE, Arend WP. Levels of synovial fluid interleukin-1 receptor antagonist in rheumatoid arthritis and other arthopathies. Arthritis Rheum 1993;36:781-9.
7. Ojo-Amaize EA, Lawless OA, Peter JB. Elevated concentrations of interleukin-1β and interleukin-1 receptor antagonist in plasma of women with silicone breast implants. Clin Diagn Lab Immun 1996;3:257-9.
8. Donnelly SC, Strieter RM, Reid PT, et al. The association between mortality rates and decreased concentrations of interleukin-10 and interleukin-1 receptor antagonist in the lung fluids of patients with adult respiratory distress syndrome. Ann Intern Med 1996;125:191-6.

Interleukin 2

Vellalore N. Kakanaiah, Ph.D.

Interleukin 2 (IL-2), a pleiotrophic lymphokine secreted primarily by activated CD4$^+$ T lymphocytes, and some CD8$^+$ T cells and B cells,[1] is a central facilitator of the immune response by supporting T-cell proliferation, augmenting natural killer (NK) cell cytotoxicity, inducing lymphokine-activated killer cell (LAK) development and participating in the activation of monocytes and B lymphocytes.[2] Production of IL-2 is altered or impaired in a variety of immunodeficiency diseases (e.g., AIDS, Nezelof syndrome and SCID) and in autoimmune diseases, including systemic lupus erythematosus (SLE) and insulin-dependent diabetes mellitus.[3,4] Lymphocytes from common variable immune deficiency (CVID), idiopathic Parkinson disease and schizophrenic patients with high concentrations of anti-hippocampal antibodies produced low IL-2 concentrations after activation.[5-7] Other data suggest overproduction of IL-2 in SLE and hypothyroidism.[8,9] In chronic progressive multiple sclerosis, IL-2 concentrations are increased in serum and/or CSF;[10-12] IL-2 is bound to serum proteins.[13] IL-2 and IL-2R are increased in the serum in diffuse and limited scleroderma,[14,15] and serum IL-2 is increased in pre-eclampsia[16] and primary antiphospholipid syndrome.[17] Plasma and urinary IL-2 and plasma IL-2R concentrations are greatly increased during renal allograft rejection or cytomegalovirus infection in patients with renal allografts.[18,19] In addition to increasing their survival, decreasing autoantibody and rheumatoid factor titers and decreasing kidney and synovial pathology, infection of MRL/*lpr* mice with recombinant IL-2/vaccinia virus is said to cause decreases in the increased numbers of CD3$^+$ CD4$^+$ CD8$^+$ ("double negative") T cells which characterize these mice and patients with SLE and rheumatoid arthritis.[20] Cyclosporin A and FK 506 prevent T-cell proliferation by inhibiting a Ca^{2+}-dependent event necessary for induction of IL-2 transcription.[21]

REFERENCES

1. Rubin JT. Interleukin-2: its biology and clinical application in patients with cancer. Cancer Invest 1993;11:460-72.
2. Swain SL. Lymphokines and the immune response: the central role of interleukin-2. Curr Opin Immunol 1991;3:304-10.
3. Riegel JS, Corthesy B, Flanagan WM, Crabtree GR. Regulation of the interleukin-2 gene. In: Kishimoto T, editor. Molecular Biology and Immunology. Basel: Chem Immunol 1992;51:266-98.
4. Kroemer G, Andreu JL, Gonzalo JA, Gutierrez-Ramos JC, Martinez-A C. Adv Immunol 1991;50:147-235.
5. Fischer MB, Hauber I, Vogel E, Wolf HM, Mannhalter JW, Eibl MM. Defective interleukin-2 and interferon-γ gene expression in response to antigen in a subgroup of patients with common variable immunodeficiency. J Allergy Clin Immunol 1993;92:340-52.
6. Kluter H, Vieregge P, Stolze H, Kirchner H. Defective production of interleukin-2 in patients with idiopathic Parkinson's disease. J Neurol Sci 1995;133:134-9.
7. Yang ZW, Chengappa KNR, Shurin G, et al. An association between anti-hippocampal antibody concentration and lymphocyte production of IL-2 in patients with schizophrenia. Psychol Med 1994;24:449-55.
8. Warrington RJ. Interleukin-2 abnormalities in systemic lupus erythematosus and rheumatoid arthritis: a role for overproduction of interleukin-2 in human autoimmunity? J Rheumatol 1988;15:616-20.
9. Komorowski J. Increased interleukin-2 level in patients with primary hypothyroidism. Clin Immunol Immunopathol 1992;63:200-2.
10. Freedman MS, Muth LK, Trotter JL, Yoshizawa CN, Antel JP. Prospective serial analysis of interleukin-2 and soluble interleukin-2 receptor in relapsing-remitting multiple sclerosis. Neurology 1992;42:1596-601.
11. Peter JB, Boctor FN, Tourtellotte WW. Serum and CSF levels of IL-2, sIL-2R, TNF-α, and IL-1β in chronic progressive multiple sclerosis: expected lack of clinical utility. Neurology 1991;41:121-3.
12. Gallo P, Piccinno M, Pagni S, Tavolato B. Interleukin-2 levels in serum and cerebrospinal fluid of multiple sclerosis patients. Ann Neurol 1988; 24:795-7.
13. Trotter JL, Damico CA, Trotter AL, Collins KG, Cross AH. Interleukin-2 binding proteins in sera from normal subjects and multiple sclerosis patients. Neurology 1995;45:1971-4.
14. Kahaleh MB, LeRoy EC. Interleukin-2 in scleroderma: correlation of serum level with extent of skin involvement and disease duration. Ann Intern Med 1989;110:446-50.
15. Clements PJ, Peter JB, Agopian MS, Telian NS, Furst DE. Elevated serum levels of soluble interleukin-2 receptor, interleukin-2 and neopterin in diffuse and limited scleroderma: effect of chlorambucil. J Rheumatol 1990;17:908-10.
16. Sunder-Plassmann G, Derfler K, Wagner L, et al. Increased serum activity of interleukin-2 in patients with pre-eclampsia. J Autoimmun 1989;2:203-5.
17. Ahmed K, Khamashta MA, Vianna JL, Hughes GRV. IL-2, IL-6 and TNF levels in primary antiphospholipid syndrome. Clin Exp Rheumatol 1992;10:503-4.
18. Cornaby A, Simpson MA, Vann Rice R, Dempsey RA, Madras PN, Monaco AP. Interleukin-2 production in plasma and urine, plasma interleukin-2 receptor levels, and urine cytology as a means of monitoring renal allograft recipients. Transplant Proc 1988;20:S108-10.
19. Colvin RB, Fuller TC, MacKeen L, Kung PC, Ip SH, Cosimi AB. Plasma interleukin-2 receptor levels in renal allograft recipients. Clin Immunol Immunopathol 1987;43:273-6.

20. Gutierrez-Ramos JC, Andreu JL, Revilla Y, Vinuela E, Martinez-A C. Recovery from autoimmunity of MRL/lpr mice after infection with an interleukin-2/vaccinia recombinant virus. Nature 1990;346:271-4.
21. O'Keefe SJ, Tamura J, Kincaid RL, Tocci MJ, O'Neill EA. FK-506- and CsA-sensitive activation of the interleukin-2 promoter by calcineurin. Nature 1992;357:692-4.

Interleukin 2 Receptor

Vellalore N. Kakanaiah, Ph.D.

Interleukin 2 receptor (IL-2R) consists of at least three distinct subunits, the α chain (IL-2Rα), the β chain (IL-2Rβ) and the γ chain (IL-2Rγ).[1] Soluble IL-2R (sIL-2R; previously known as Tac) is the released extracellular domain of the IL-2Rα (low affinity, p55) by activated cells (probably including T cells, B cells and macrophages) during a variety of immune responses[2] including rheumatoid arthritis (RA), ankylosing spondylitis, systemic lupus erythematosus, scleroderma, myositis, host-versus-graft reaction, lymphoreticular malignancies, systemic parasitic diseases, AIDS, Graves disease, inflammatory bowel disease, myasthenia gravis, chronic progressive multiple sclerosis and asthma.[3-16] In RA, sIL2R concentrations do not correlate with short-term clinical measures of disease activity after various treatments.[17-18] In other diseases (cutaneous T-cell lymphoma[19] and Guillain-Barré syndrome[20]), higher sIL-2R concentrations correlate with the disease activity; whereas, no correlation is seen in epithelial ovarian cancer patients.[21] Elevated sIL-2R concentrations are found in bile and in lower concentrations in serum of liver transplant patients before and during acute rejection episodes.[22] Serum sIL-2R concentrations increase progressively from stages I and II to stages III and IV of IgA nephropathy,[23] but the significance of this is uncertain because serum sIL-2R increases in patients with chronic renal failure.[24] Although of pathogenetic interest, none of these increases are shown to be incontrovertibly useful for evaluation of disease activity or therapeutic monitoring.[25]

REFERENCES
1. Minami Y, Kono T, Miyazaki T, Taniguchi T. The IL-2 receptor complex: its structure, function, and target genes. Annu Rev Immunol 1993;11:245-67.
2. Obara T, Vodian MA, Kung PC. Clinical significance of soluble interleukin-2 receptor for monitoring the diseases associated with activated lymphocytes and viral infections. J Clin Lab Anal 1992;6:423-36.
3. Wolf RE, Brelsford WG, Hall VC, Adams SB. Cytokines and soluble interleukin-2 receptors in rheumatoid arthritis. J Rheumatol 1992;19:524-8.
4. Wendling D, Racadot E, Viel JF. Soluble interleukin-2 receptor in patients with ankylosing spondylitis. Arthritis Rheum 1991;34:1622-3.
5. Sawada S, Hashimoto H, Iijma S, et al. Increased soluble IL-2 receptor in serum of patients with systemic lupus erythematosus. Clin Rheumatol 1993;12:204-9.
6. Peter JB, Agopian MS, Clements PJ, Telian NS, Furst DE. Elevated serum levels of interleukin-2 receptor (IL-2R) and IL-2 in diffuse (DS) and limited scleroderma (LS) [Abstract]. J Rheumatol 1990;17:908-10.
7. Tokano Y, Kanai Y, Hashimoto H, Okumura K, Hirose S. Soluble interleukin-2 receptors in patients with polymyositis/dermatomyositis. Ann Rheum Dis 1992;51:781-2.
8. Carlson IH. New markers in serum for lymphocyte activation for predicting allograft rejection. Neopterin and soluble interleukin-2 receptors. Clin Lab Med 1992;12:99-111.
9. Pavlidis NA, Manoussakis MN, Germanidis GS, Moutsopoulos HM. Serum-soluble interleukin-2 receptors in B-cell lymphoproliferative malignancies. Med Pediatr Oncol 1992;20:26-31.
10. Josimovic-Alasevic O, Feldmeier H, Zwingenberger K, et al. Interleukin-2 receptor in patients with localized and systemic parasitic diseases. Clin Exp Immunol 1988;72:249-54.
11. Noronha IL, Daniel V, Schimpf K, Opelz G. Soluble IL-2 receptor and tumour necrosis factor-alpha in plasma of haemophilia patients infected with HIV. Clin Exp Immunol 1992;87:287-92.
12. Prummel MF, Wiersinga WM, Van der Gaag R, Mourtis MP, Koornneef L. Soluble IL-2 receptor levels in patients with Graves' ophthalmopathy. Clin Exp Immunol 1992;88:405-9.
13. Matsuura T, West GA, Klein JS, Ferraris L, Fiocchi C. Soluble interleukin-2 and CD8 and CD4 receptors in inflammatory bowel disease. Gastroenterology 1992;102:2006-14.
14. Cohen-Kaminsky S, Jacques Y, Aime C, Safar D, Morel E, Berrih-Aknin S. Follow-up of soluble interleukin-2 receptor levels after thymectomy in patients with myasthenia gravis. Clin Immunol Immunopathol 1992;62:190-8.
15. Peter JB, Boctor FN, Tourtellotte WW. Serum and CSF levels of IL-2, sIL-2R, TNF-α, and IL-1β in chronic progressive multiple sclerosis: expected lack of clinical utility. Neurology 1991;41:121-3.

16. Motojima S, Hirata A, Kishima A, et al. Serum levels of soluble interleukin-2 receptor in asthma patients. J Asthma 1995;32:151-8.
17. Portioli I. Serum soluble interleukin-2 receptor levels in rheumatoid arthritis: correlation with clinical and immunological parameters and with the response to auranofin treatment. Clin Exp Rheumatol 1994;12:357-62.
18. Pollison RP, Dooley MA, Dawson DV, Pisetsky DS. Interleukin-2 receptor levels in the sera of rheumatoid arthritis patients treated with methotrexate. Arthritis Rheum 1994;37:50-6.
19. Wasik MA, Vonderheid EC, Bigler RD, et al. Increased serum concentrations of the soluble interleukin-2 receptor in cutaneous T-cell lymphoma. Arch Dermatol 1996;132:42-7.
20. Bansil S, Mithen FA, Cook SD, Sheffet A, Rohowsky-Kochan C. Clinical correlation with serum-soluble interleukin-2 receptor levels in Guillain-Barré syndrome. Neurology 1991;41:1302-5.
21. Pavlidis NA, Bairaktari E, Kalef-Ezra J, Nicolaides C, Seferiadis C, Fountzilas G. Serum soluble interleukin-2 receptors in epithelial ovarian cancer patients. Int J Biol Markers 1995;10:75-80.
22. Adams DH, Wang L, Hubscher SG, Elias E, Neuberger JM. Soluble interleukin-2 receptors in serum and bile of liver transplant recipients. Lancet 1989;1:469-71.
23. Tomino Y, Ozaki T, Koide H, Takahashi M, Ito K. Serum levels of interleukin-2 receptor and disease activity in patients with IgA nephropathy. J Clin Lab Analysis 1989;3:355-9.
24. Takamatsu T, Yasuda N, Ohno T, et al. Soluble interleukin-2 receptors in the serum of patients with chronic renal failure. Tohoku J Exp Med 1988;155:343-7.
25. Schroeder TJ, Helling T, McKenna RM, et al. A multicenter study to evaluate a novel assay for quantitation of soluble interleukin-2 receptor in renal transplant recipients. Transplantation 1992;53:34-40.

Interleukin 3

Vellalore N. Kakanaiah, Ph.D.

Interleukin 3 (IL-3), a pluripotent hematopoietic growth factor produced primarily by activated T cells, stimulates proliferation, differentiation, and function of multipotential hematopoietic stem cells and committed progenitor cells of granulocytes, macrophages, megakaryocytes, mast cells and erythroid cell lineages.[1] In autologous bone marrow transplantation patients, combined treatment with IL-3 and G-CSF causes rapid hematopoietic recovery following myeloablative chemotherapy.[2] IL-3 and GM-CSF might be important in the pathogenesis of acute severe asthma through their regulatory role on eosinophil survival, differentiation and effector function.[3] IL-3 indirectly enhances the activity of cytotoxic T cells by stimulating the release of T-cell growth factors in experimental systems.[4]

REFERENCES
1. Lindermann A, Mertelsmann R. Interleukin-3 and its receptor. Cancer Treat Res 1995;80:107-42.
2. Lemoli RM, Rosti G, Visani G, et al. Concomitant and sequential administration of recombinant human granulocyte colony-stimulating factor and recombinant human interleukin-3 to accelerate hematopoietic recovery after autologous bone marrow transplantation for malignant lymphoma. J Clin Oncol 1996;14:3018-25.
3. Lai CK, Ho SS, Chan Ch, Leung R, Lai KN. Gene expression of interleukin-3 and granulocyte macrophage colony-stimulating factor in circulating CD4+ T cells in acute severe asthma. Clin Exp Allergy 1996;26:138-46.
4. Pulaski BA, McAdam AJ, Hutter EK, Bigger S, Lord EM, Frelinger JG. IL-3 enhances development of tumor reactive cytotoxic cells by a CD4 dependent mechanism. Cancer Res 1993;53:2112-7.

Interleukin 4

Vellalore N. Kakanaiah, Ph.D.

Interleukin 4 (IL-4, previously known as B-cell growth factor) is primarily produced by activated helper T cells and mast cells.[1] IL-4 affects a variety of cell types, including B and T lymphocytes, natural killer cells, lymphokine-activated killer cells, monocytes/macrophages, mast cells, eosinophils, basophils, fibroblasts, endothelial cells, and various human tumors of hematopoietic and nonhematopoietic origin.[1,2] IL-4 is an autocrine factor for murine T_H2 cell lines.[2] IL-4 enhances the proliferation and differentiation of CTL precursors,[3] and *in vitro* exerts anti-tumor responses in some hematopoietic tumor cells.[1,4] In mice, IL-4 mediates Ig class switching to produce IgE.[2] The fact that glucocorticoids increase synthesis of IgE by human lymphocytes in the presence of IL-4 might explain the increase in IgE production in steroid-treated allergic patients and the increased production of IgE after stress, e.g., myocardial infraction.[5] B cells from SLE patients,[6] and CD4[+] T cells infiltrating skin lesions of patients with atopic dermatitis, produce higher levels of IL-4.[7] IL-4 is not increased in rheumatoid arthritis synovial fluid.[8] Administration of IL-4 can induce serious adverse reactions *in vivo*, which include mild fever, headache, sinus congestion, nausea and elevated hepatic enzymes.[1]

REFERENCES
1. Puri RK, Siegel JP. Interleukin-4 and cancer therapy. Cancer Invest 1993:11:473-86.
2. Paul WE. Interleukin-4: a prototypic immunoregulatory lymphokine. Blood 1990:77:1859-70.
3. Trenn G, Takayama H, Hu-Li J, Paul WE, Sitkovsky MV. B cell stimulatory factor 1 (IL-4) enhances the development of cytotoxic T cells from Lyt2+ resting murine T lymphocytes. J Immunol 1988:140:1101-8.
4. Tepper RI, Coffman RL, Leder P. An eosinophil-dependent mechanism for the antitumor effect of IL-4. Science 1992:257:548-51.
5. Wu CY, Sarfati M, Heusser C, et al. Glucocorticoids increase the synthesis of immunoglobulin E by interleukin 4 stimulated human lymphocytes. J Clin Invest 1991:87:870-7.
6. Tanaka Y, Saito K, Shirakawa F, et al. Production of B-cell stimulatory factors by B cells in patients with systemic lupus erythematosus. J Immunol 1988:141:3043-9.
7. van der Heijden FL, Wierenga EA, Bos JD, et al. High frequency of IL-4 producing CD4[+] allergen-specific T lymphocytes in atopic dermatitis lesional skin. J Invest Dermatol 1991:97:389-94.
8. Miossec P, Naviliat M, D'Angeac AD, Sany J, Banchereau J. Low levels of interleukin-4 and high levels of transforming growth factor b in rheumatoid synovitis. Arthritis Rheum 1990;33:1180-8.

Interleukin 5

Vellalore N. Kakanaiah, Ph.D.

Interleukin 5 (IL-5), which is produced by activated T cells, mast cells, and eosinophils,[1,2] is a critical cytokine associated with eosinophil and lymphocyte recruitement into the airways of patients with asthma following exposure to allergen.[3] IL-5 is a more restricted hematopoietic growth factor than IL-3. IL-5 controls the eosinophil and basophil lineages.[4] Expression of IL-5 by Reed-Sternberg cells suggests a T-cell origin for these cells and might explain the eosinophilia in Hodgkin disease.[5] However, there could be species differences. In mice, IL-5 (like IL-4 which stimulates IgE responses) is produced by the T_H2 subset of CD4[+] T-cell lines; addition of MAb to IL-5 inhibits helminth-induced eosinophilia in bone marrow, peripheral blood, and in the egg granulomas of acute schistosomiasis.[6]

REFERENCES
1. Sanderson CJ, Campbell HD, Young IG. Molecular and cellular biology of eosinophil differentiation factor (interleukin-5) and its effects on human and mouse B cells. Immunol Rev 1988;102:29.
2. Lamkhioued B, Gounni AS, Aldebert D, et al. Synthesis of type 1 (IFN-γ) and type 2 (IL-4, IL-5, and IL-10) cytokines by human eosinophils. Ann N Y Acad Sci 1996;796:203-8.
3. Sur S, Gleich GJ, Offord KP, et al. Allergen challenge in asthma: association of eosinophils and lymphocytes with interleukin-5. Allergy 1995;50:891-8.
4. Lopez AF, Elliott MG, Woodock J, Vadas MA. GM-CSF, IL-3 and IL-5: Cross-competition on human haemopoietic cells. Immunol Today 1992;13:495-8.
5. Samoszuk M, Nansen L. Detection of interleukin-5 messenger RNA in Reed-Sternberg cells of Hodgkin's disease with eosinophilia. Blood 1990;75:13-6.
6. Sher A, Coffman RL, Hieny S, Scott P, Cheever AW. Interleukin 5 is required for the blood and tissue eosinophilia but not granuloma formation induced by infection with *Schistosoma mansoni*. Proc Natl Acad Sci USA 1990;87:61-5.

Interleukin 6

Vellalore N. Kakanaiah, Ph.D.

Interleukin 6 (IL-6), originally identified as a B-cell stimulator factor-2 (BSF-2), is a pleiotropic cytokine that acts not only on B cells but also on T cells, hepatocytes, hematopoietic progenitor cells and neuronal cells.[1] IL-6 is important in acute phase reactions and is expressed by a variety of normal and transformed cells including T cells, B cells, monocytes/macrophages, fibroblasts, hepatocytes, keratinocytes, astrocytes, vascular endothelial cells, mesangial cells, osteoblasts, Sertoli cells, carcinomas, sarcomas, myelomas, glioblatomas and melanomas.[1-3] The pleiotropic functions of IL-6 are summarized below (Table).[1] IL-6 is associated with hyperglobulinemia and autoantibody production when secreted by cardiac myxomas or cervical carcinomas.[4] IL-6 is elevated post-operatively[5] in infection/community-acquired pneumonia,[6,7] in alcoholic hepatitis[8] and in chronic renal failure.[9]

In endotoxin-induced uveitis in rats, which is a model for the uveitis of seronegative spondylarthritis, aqueous-human level of IL-6 was tenfold than seen in serum suggesting intraocular synthesis of IL-6.[10] IL-6 is increased in serum of children with Still disease, in synovial fluid and sometimes in serum in rheumatoid arthritis (RA), in CSF of patients with bacterial meningitis as well as in CNS-lupus, in paraneoplastic syndrome (occasionally found with pheochromocytoma) and in Castleman disease/POEMS.[11-18] In RA, as well as in multiple myeloma, there is no useful correlation between IL-6 concentrations and prognosis/diagnosis during treatment regimes.[13,14,19,20] IL-6 concentrations are higher in SLE patients compared to RA patients,[21] but in some SLE patients, lower IL-6 concentrations may be due to the presence of IL-6 antibodies and soluble IL-6 receptor.[22] IL-6 is a co-stimulus for con A activation of purified T cells.[23] IL-6 is also detected in urine from patients with a variety of renal lesions,[24] and is increased in patients with nephropathia epidemia; a European form of hantavirus-induced hemorrhagic fever with renal syndrome.[25] Release of IL-6 by normal and neoplastic B cells and by cells derived from AIDS Kaposi sarcomas[26] is expected to have important effects on cells in their microenvironment.[27] Serum IL-6 concentrations correlate with disease severity in plasma cell dyscrasias.[28] Plasma (EDTA and aprotinin) is probably more appropriate for study than serum.[29] IL-6 is increased in plasma and on dermal and epidermal cells in lesional skin of psoriasis.[30] Increases of serum IL-6 are found in Castleman disease,[31] in which inappropriate synthesis of IL-6 probably has a primary role in pathogenesis.[32] IL-6 is increased in CSF in ~50% of HTLV-I-associated myelopathy and in about 80% (12/15) of amyotrophic lateral sclerosis.[33] Treatment with antibodies to IL-6 prevents the hypergammaglobulinemia of experimental cerebral malaria.[34] Increased post-menopausal osteoclast development is stimulated by IL-6 and inhibited by estrogens,[35] plasma IL-6 concentrations are elevated in post-menopausal women.[36]

Pleiotropic Effects of IL-6	
B cells	Ig production Proliferation of myeloma cells Proliferation of Epstein-Barr virus-infected B cells
T cells	Proliferation and differentiation of T cells Differentiation of cytotoxic T lymphocytes Induction of IL-2R expression and IL-2 production Augmentation of NK activities
Hematopoietic progenitor cells	Enhancement of multipotential hematopoietic colony formation
Megakaryocytes	Megakaryocyte maturation
Macrophages	Growth inhibition of myeloid leukemic cells lines and induction of their macrophage differentiation
Hepatocytes	Acute-phase protein synthesis
Bone metabolism	Stimulation of osteoclast formation Induction of bone resorption
Blood vessels	Induction of platelet-derived growth factor Proliferation of vascular smooth muscle cells

Pleiotropic Effects of IL-6	
Heart muscle cells	Negative inotropic effect on heart
Neuronal cells	Neural differentiation of PC12 cells
	Support of survival of cholinergic neurons
	Induction of adrenocorticotropic hormone synthesis
Placenta	Secretion of chorionic gonadotropin from trophoblasts

Modified from Kishimoto T, et al. Blood 1995;86:1243-54.

REFERENCES

1. Kishimoto T, Akira S, Narazaki M, Taga T. Interleukin-6 family of cytokines and gp130. Blood 1995;86:1243-54.
2. Hirano T. The biology of interleukin-6. In: Kishimoto T, editor. Interleukins: Molecular Biology and Immunology. Basel: Chem Immunol 1992;51:153-80.
3. Bauer J, Herrmann F. Interleukin-6 in clinical medicine. Ann Hematol 1991;62:203-10.
4. Jourdan M, Bataille R, Seguin J, Zhang XG, Chaptal PA, Klein B. Constitutive production of interleukin-6 and immunologic features in cardiac myxomas. Arthritis Rheum 1990;33:398-402.
5. Ohzato H, Yoshizaki K, Nishimoto N, et al. Interleukin-6 as a new indicator of inflammatory status: detection of serum levels of interleukin-6 and C-reactive protein after surgery. Surgery 1992;111:201-9.
6. Chen Y-M, Whang-Peng J, Chen C-H, Kuo BI-T, Wang S-Y, Perng R-P. Elevation of serum IL-6 levels in patients with acute bacterial infection. Chin Med J 1995;56:239-43.
7. Örtqvist C, Hedlund J, Wretlind B, Carlstr`m A, Kalin M. Diagnostic and prognostic value of interleukin-6 and C-reactive protein in community-acquired pneumonia. Scand J Infect Dis 1995;27:457-62.
8. Hill DB, Marsano L, Cohen D, Allen J, Shedlofsky S, McClain CJ. Increased plasma interleukin-6 concentrations in alcoholic hepatitis. J Lab Clin Med 1992;119:547-52.
9. Herbelin A, Ureña P, Nguyen AT, Zingraff J, Descamps-Latscha B. Elevated circulating levels of interleukin-6 in patients with chronic renal failure. Kidney Int 1991;39:954-60.
10. Hoekzema R, Murray PI, van Haren MAC, Helle M, Kijlstra A. Analysis of interleukin-6 in endotoxin-induced uveitis. Invest Ophthalmol Vis Sci 1991;32:88-95.
11. Kishimoto T. Factors affecting B-cell growth and differentiation. Annu Rev Immunol 1985;3:133-57.
12. Brozik M, Rosztóczy I, Merétey K, et al. Interleukin 6 levels in synovial fluids of patients with different arthritides: correlation with local IgM rheumatoid factor and systemic acute phase protein production. J Rheumatol 1992;19:63-8.
13. Wascher TC, Herrman J, Brezinschek R, et al. Serum levels of interleukin-6 and tumor-necrosis factor-alpha are not correlated to disease activity in patients with rheumatoid arthritis after treatment with low-dose methotrexate. Eur J Clin Invest 1994;24:73-5.
14. Cohick CB, Furst DE, Quagliata S, et al. Analysis of elevated serum interleukin-6 levels in rheumatoid arthritis: correlation with erythrocyte sedimentation rate or C-reactive protein. J Lab Clin Med 1994;123:721-7.
15. Rusconi F, Parizzi F, Garlaschi L, et al. Interleukin 6 activity in infants and children with bacterial meningitis. Pediatr Infect Dis J 1991;10:117-21.
16. Hirohata S, Miyamoto T. Elevated levels of Interleukin-6 in cerebrospinal fluid from patients with systemic lupus erythematosus and central nervous system involvement. Arthritis Rheum 1990;33:644-9.
17. Fukumoto S, Matsumoto T, Harada S-I, Fujisaki J, Kawano M, Ogata E. Pheochromocytoma with pyrexia and marked inflammatory signs: a paraneoplastic syndrome with possible relation to interleukin-6 production. J Clin Endocrinol Metab 1991;73:877-81.
18. Mandler RN, Kerrigan DP, Smart J, Kuis W, Villiger P, Lotz M. Castleman's disease in POEMS syndrome with elevated interleukin-6. Cancer 1992;69:2697-2703.
19. Tharasu PW, Ganjoo RK, Maidment SA, et al. Multiple myeloma: an immunoclinical study of disease and response to treatment. Hematol Oncol 1995;13:69-82.
20. Kyrstsonis M-C, Dedoussis G, Baxevanis C, Stamatelous M, Maniatis A. Serum interleukin-6 (IL-6) and interleukin-4 (IL-4) in patients with multiple myeloma (MM). Br J Haematol 1996;92:420-2.
21. Gabay C, Roux-Lombard P, de Moerloose P, Dayer J-M, Vischer T, Guerne P-A. Absence of correlation between interleukin-6 and C-reactive protein blood levels in systemic lupus erythematosus compared with rheumatoid arthritis. J Rheumatol 1993;20:815-21.
22. Evans M, Abdou NI. Anti-interleukin-6 and soluble interleukin-6 receptor in systemic lupus erythematosus. Lupus 1994;3:161-6.
23. Garman RD, Jacobs KA, Clark SC, Raulet DH. B-cell stimulatory factor 2 (β_2 interferon) functions as a second signal for interleukin 2 production by mature murine T cells. Proc Natl Acad Sci USA 1987;84:7629-33.

24. Gordon C, Richards N, Howie AJ, et al. Urinary IL-6: a marker for mesangial proliferative glomerulonephritis? Clin Exp Immunol 1991;86:145-9.
25. Linderholm M, Ahlm C, Settergren B, Waage A, Tärnvik A. Elevated plasma levels of tumor necrosis factor (TNF)-I, soluble TNF receptors, interleukin (IL)-6, and IL-10 in patients with hemorrhagic fever with renal syndrome. J Infect Dis 1996;173:38-43.
26. Miles SA, Rezai AR, Salazar-González JF, et al. AIDS Kaposi sarcoma-derived cells produce and respond to interleukin-6. Proc Natl Acad Sci USA 1990;87:4068-72.
27. Freeman GJ, Freedman AS, Rabinowe SN, et al. Interleukin-6 gene expression in normal and neoplastic B cells. J Clin Invest 1989;83:1512-8.
28. Solary E, Guiguet M, Zeller V, et al. Radioimmunoassay for the measurement of serum IL-6 and its correlation with tumour cell mass parameters in multiple myeloma. Am J Hematol 1992;39:163-71.
29. Cannon JG, van der Meer JWM, Kwiatkowski D, et al. Interleukin-1J in human plasma: optimization of blood collection, plasma extraction, and radioimmunoassay methods. Lymphokine Res 1988;7:457-67.
30. Grossman RM, Krueger J, Yourish D, et al. Interleukin-6 is expressed in high levels in psoriatic skin and stimulates proliferation of cultured human keratinocytes. Proc Natl Acad Sci USA 1989;86:6367-71.
31. Hsu S-M, Xie S-S, Hsu P-L, Waldron JA Jr. Interleukin-6, but not interleukin-4, is expressed by Reed-Sternberg cells in Hodgkin's disease with or without histologic features of Castleman's disease. Am J Pathol 1992;141:129-38.
32. Brandt SJ, Bodine DM, Dunbar CE, Nienhus AW. Dysregulated interleukin-6 expression produces a syndrome resembling Castleman's disease in mice. J Clin Invest 1990;86:592-9.
33. Ohbo K, Sugamura K, Sekizawa T, Kogure K. Interleukin-6 in cerebrospinal fluid of HTLV-I-associated myelopathy. Neurology 1991;41:594-5.
34. Grau GE, Frei K, Piguet P-F, et al. Interleukin-6 production in experimental cerebral malaria: modulation by anticytokine antibodies and possible role in hypergammaglobulinemia. J Exp Med 1990;172:1505-8.
35. Jilka RL, Hangoc G, Girasole G, et al. Increased osteoclast development after estrogen loss: mediation by interleukin-6. Science 1992;257:88-91.
36. Kania DM, Binkley N, Checovich M, Harighurst T, Schilling M, Ershler WB. Elevated plasma levels of interleukin-6 in postmenopausal women do not correlate with bone density. J Am Geriatr Soc 1995;43:236-9.

Interleukin 7

Vellalore N. Kakanaiah, Ph.D.

Interleukin 7 (IL-7, originally known as lymphopoietin-1), which is produced by bone marrow stromal cells and supports growth of pre-B cells in the absence of other cytokines or stromal cells,[1] is a growth factor for immature and mature thymocytes and interacts with other cytokines in the thymus to regulate proliferation and differentiation of thymocytes.[2] In short-term cultures, human peripheral blood T cells proliferate in response to IL-7 when combined with CD3 antibodies or lectin. In long-term cultures, however, IL-7 alone is sufficient to promote growth.[2,3] IL-7 enhances the cytotoxic activity of human CD8[+] CTL stimulated with ConA and IL-2 or antigen.[4] IL-7 also increases LAK activity of NK-cells independently of IL-2,[5] is a potent growth factor for both Sezary[6] and T acute lymphoblastic leukemia cells,[6,7] and upregulates HIV-1 replication in naturally infected PBMCs in culture.[8] Elevated plasma IL-7 concentrations are found in patients with systemic juvenile rheumatoid arthritis and are associated with the presence and severity of systemic symptoms.[9]

REFERENCES
1. Appasamy PM. Interleukin-7 and lymphopoiesis: biological and clinical implications. Cancer Treat Res 1995;80:235-60.
2. Appasamy PM. Interleukin-7: biology and potential clinical applications. Cancer Investigation 1993;11:487-99.
3. Morrissey PJ, Goodwin RG, Nordan RP, et al. Recombinant interleukin-7, pre-B cell growth factor, has costimulatory activity on purified mature T cells. J Exp Med 1989;169:707-16.
4. Hickman CJ, Crim JA, Mostowski HS, et al. Regulation of human cytotoxic T lymphocyte development by IL-7. J Immunol 1990;145:2415-20.
5. Dadmarz R, Bockstoce DC, Golub SH. Interleukin-7 selectively enhances natural kill cytotoxicity mediated by the CD56[bright] natural killer subpopulation. Lymphokine Cytokine Res 1994;13:349-57.
6. Merle-Béral H, Schmitt C, Mossalayi D, Bismuth G, Dalloul A, Mentz F. Interleukin-7 and malignant T cells. Nouv Rev Fr Hematol 1993;35:231-2.

7. Eder M, Hemmati P, Kalina U, et al. Effects of Flt3 ligand and interleukin-7 on in vitro growth of acute lymphoblastic leukemic cells. Exp Hematol 1996;24:371-7.
8. Smithgall MD, Wong JG, Critchett KE, Haffer OK. IL-7 up-regulates HIV-1 replication in naturally infected peripheral blood mononuclear cells. J Immunol 1996;156:2324-30.
9. De Benedetti F, Massa M, Pignatti P, et al. Elevated circulating interleukin-7 levels in patients with systemic juvenile rheumatoid arthritis. J Rheumatol 1995;22:1581-5.

Interleukin 8

Vellalore N. Kakanaiah, Ph.D.

Interleukin 8 (IL-8, previously known as neutrophil-activating peptide, NAP-1), which belongs to a family of chemoattractants, is produced by monocytes, macrophages, T cells, NK cells and a variety of non-lymphoid cell types in response to IL-1 or TNF-α, as well as mitogens, lectins, phorbol esters and viruses.[1,2] IL-8 causes T cell, basophil and neutrophil activation, chemotaxis and edema. IL-8 is detectable in psoriatic scales,[3] synovial fluid of patients with RA[4] or gout,[5] pleural fluid from emphysema patients,[6] alvelolar macrophages from lungs with idiopathic pulmonary fibrosis,[7] broncheoalveolar lavage fluids from patients with adult respiratory distress syndrome,[8] cystic fibrosis,[9] chronic bronchitis[1] and diffuse panbronchiolitis.[10] IL-8 is also detectable in patients with severe bacterial infections, septicemia,[11] chronic sarcoidosis,[12] alcoholic hepatitis[13] and HIV infection.[14]

REFERENCES
1. Hébert CA, Baker JB. Interleukin-8: a review. Cancer Invest 1993;11:743-50.
2. Hoch RC, Schraufstatter IU, Cochrane CG. In vivo, in vitro, and molecular aspects of interleukin-8 and the interleukin-8 receptors. J Lab Clin Med 1996;128:134-45.
3. Konstantinova NV, Duong DM, Remenyik E, Hazarika P, et al. Interleukin-8 is induced in skin equivalents and is highest in those derived from psoriatic fibroblasts. J Invest Dermatol 1996;107:615-21.
4. Koch A, Kunkel S, Burrows J, et al. Synovial tissue macrophages as a source of the chemotactic cytokine IL-8. J Immunol 1991;147:2187-95.
5. Terkeltaub R, Zachariae C, Santoro D, et al. Monocyte-derived neutrophil chemotactic factor/interleukin-8 is a potential mediator of crystal-induced inflammation. Arthritis Rheum 1991;34:894-903.
6. Broaddus V, Hébert C, Vitangcol R, et al. Interleukin-8 is a major neutrophil chemotactic factor in pleural liquid of patients with emphysema. Am Rev Respir Dis 1992;146:825-30.
7. Carré P, Mortenson R, King T, et al. Increased expression of the interleukin-8 gene by alveolar macrophages in idiopathic pulmonary fibrosis. J Clin Invest 1991;88:1802-10.
8. Miller EJ, Cohen AB, Nagao S, et al. Elevated levels of NAP-1/Interleukin-8 are present in the airspaces of patients with adult respiratory distress syndrome and are associated with increased mortality. Am Rev Resp Dis 1992;146:427-32.
9. McElvaney N, Nakamura H, Birrer P, et al. Modulation of airway inflammation in cystic fibrosis: in vivo suppression of interleukin-8 levels on the respiratory epithelial surface by aerosolization of recombinant secretory leukoprotease inhibitor. J Clin Invest 1992;90:1296-1301.
10. Sakito O, Kadota J, Kohno S, et al. Interleukin 1 beta, tumor necrosis factor alpha, and interleukin 8 in bronchoalveolar lavage fluid of patients with diffuse panbronchiolitis: a potential mechanism of macrolide therapy. Respiration 1996;63:42-8.
11. Kunkel SL, Lukacs NW, Strieter RM. The role of interleukin-8 in the infectious process. Ann N Y Acad Sci 1994;730:134-43.
12. Yokoyama T, Kanda T, Kobayashi I, Suzuki T. Serum levels of interleukin-8 as a marker of disease activity in patients with chronic sarcoidosis. J Med 1995;26:209-19.
13. Huang YS, Chan CY, Wu JC, et al. Serum levels of interleukin-8 in alcoholic liver disease: relationship with disease stage, biochemical parameters and survival. J Hepatol 1996;24:377-84.
14. Matsumoto T, Miike T, Nelson RP, Trudeau WL, Lockey RF, Yodoi J. Elevated seruml levels of IL-8 in patients with HIV infection. Clin Exp Immunol 1993;93:149-51.

Interleukin 9

Vellalore N. Kakanaiah, Ph.D.

Interleukin 9 (IL-9) is a multifunctional cytokine produced by T cells after activation by either lectin or CD3 antibodies.[1] Antibodies to IL-2 completely block the cytokine-cascade-induced expression of IL-9 by activated T cells.[2] IL-9 stimulates the proliferation of primitive hematopoietic erythroid and pluripotent progenitor cells, as well as the growth of selected colony-stimulating factor-dependent myeloid cell lines.[3] IL-9 is actively involved in mast cell responses by inducing the proliferation and differentiation of these cells,[1] and can also synergize with IL-4 to induce IgE and IgG production or IgG and IgM production by B cells.[4]

REFERENCES
1. Renauld JC, Kermouni A, Vink A, Louahed J, Van Snick J. Interleukin-9 and its receptor: involvement in mast cell differentiation and T cell oncogenesis. J Leuko Biol 1995;57:353-60.
2. Houssiau FA, Schandene L, Stevens M, et al. A cascade of cytokine is responsible for IL-9 expression in human T cells. Involvement of IL-2, IL-4, and IL-10. J Immunol 1995;154:2624-30.
3. Lemoli RM, Fortuna A, Tafuri A, et al. Interleukin-9 stimulates the proliferation of human myeloid leukemic cells. Blood 1996;87:3852-9.
4. Renauld JC, Houssiau F, Druez, C. Interleukin-9. Int Rev Exp Pathol 1993;34A:99-109.

Interleukin 10

Vellalore N. Kakanaiah, Ph.D.

Interleukin 10 (IL-10, originally known as cytokine synthesis inhibitory factor), a pleiotropic cytokine produced by activated subpopulations of T cells, B cells, monocytes/macrophages, keratinocytes and tumor cells,[1] is a potent inhibitor of cell-mediated immune responses by preferential action on antigen-presenting cells.[1] IL-10 inhibits both the expression of class II MHC molecules and the production by human monocytes *in vitro* of proinflammatory cytokines such as IL-1, IL-6, IL-8, TNF-I and GM-CSF.[1,2] In contrast, IL-1 has a stimulatory effect on humoral immune responses.[3,4] IL-10 induces secretion of IgG, IgM and IgA by activated B cells and with IL-4 induces secretion of IgE.[5] Similarly, hyperactivity of B cells in SLE results from the combination of IL-10-mediated autocrine and paracrine stimulations.[6]

In rheumatoid arthritis, synovial membrane cells spontaneously produce IL-10[7] and activated T-cell clones from rheumatoid synovial membrane produce high levels of IL-10.[8] In this way, IL-10 acts as an antiinflammatory cytokine.[9] IL-10 can be detected in patients with septicemia, and there is a significant association between admission hypotension and the presence of IL-10 in severely injured patients.[10,11] IL-10 concentrations are elevated in both serum and CSF of children with bacterial meningitis.[12,13]

REFERENCES
1. Goldman M, Velu T. Interleukin-10 and its implications for immunopathology. Adv Nephrol 1995;24:79-90.
2. De Waal Malefyt R, Abrams J, Bennett B, Fidgor CG, de Vries JE. Interleukin-10 (IL-10) inhibits cytokine synthesis by human monocytes: an autoregulatory role of IL-10 produced by monocytes. J Exp Med 1991;174:1209-20.
3. Rousset F, Garcia E, Defrance T, et al. Interleukin-10 is a potent growth and differentiation factor for activated human lymphocytes-B. Proc Natl Acad Sci USA 1992;89:1890-3.
4. Benjamin D, Park CD, Sharma V. Human B cell interleukin 10. Leuk Lymphoma 1994;12:205-10.
5. Rousset F, Garcia E, Defrance T, et al. Interleukin 10 is a potent growth and differentiation factor for activated human B lymphocytes. Proc Natl Acad Sci USA 1992;89:1980-3.
6. Llorente L, Zou W, Levy Y, et al. Role of interleukin 10 in the B lymphocyte hyperactivity and autoantibody production of human systemic lupus erythematosus. J Exp Med 1995;181:839-44
7. Katsikis PD, Chu C-Q, Brennan FM, Maini RN, Fedlmann M. Immunoregulatory role of interleukin 10 in rheumatoid arthritis. J Exp Med 1994;179:1517-27.
8. Cohen SBA, Katsikis PD, Chu C-Q, et al. High level of interleukin-10 production by the activated T cell population within the rheumatoid synovial membrane. Arthritis Rheum 1995;38:946-52.
9. Isomäki P, Luukkainen R, Saario R, Toivanen P, Punnonen J. Interleukin-10 functions as an antiinflammatory cytokine in rheumatoid synovium. Arthritis Rheum 1996;39:386-95.
10. Merchant A, Deviere J, Baudouin B, et al. Interleukin-10 production during septicemia. Lancet 1994;343:707.
11. Sherry RM, Cue JI, Goddard JK, Parramore JB, DiPiro JT. Interleukin-10 is associated with the development of sepsis in trauma patients. J Trauma 1996;40:613-6.

12. van Furth AM, Seijimonsbergen EM, Langerman JAM, Groeneveld PHP, de Bel CE, van Furth R. High levels of interleukin 10 and tumor necrosis factor I in cerebrospinal fluid during the onset of bacterial meningitis. Clin Infect Dis 1995;21:220-2.
13. Kornelisse RF, Savelkoul HFJ, Mulder PHG, et al. Interleukin-10 and soluble tumor necrosis factor receptors in cerebrospinal fluid of children with bacterial meningitis. J Infect Dis 1996;173:1498-1502.

Interleukin 11

Vellalore N. Kakanaiah, Ph.D.

Interleukin 11 (IL-11), a pleiotropic cytokine which acts on hematopoietic, hepatic, stromal, epithelial, neural and osteoclast cells,[1] enhances the growth of early progenitors and promoters of megakaryocytopoiesis and erythropoiesis in *in vitro* cultures. Administration to healthy animals stimulates megakaryocyte maturation and increases peripheral platelet counts.[2] IL-11 in combination with IL-3, provides a radioprotective effect and can enhance recovery of platelets, WBC, and RBC in irradiated mice.[3] IL-11 therapy significantly decreases the morbidity and mortality due to chemotherapy-related endogenous infections. This radioprotective effect of IL-11 is mediated, at least in part, via the modulation of TNF poduction.[4]

REFERENCES
1. Yanc C. Interleukin-11 (IL-11) and its receptor: biology and potential clinical applications in thrombocytopenic states. Cancer Treat Res 1995;80:321-40.
2. Teramura M, Kobayashi S, Yoshinaga K, Iwabe K, Mizoguchi H. Effect of interleukin 11 on normal and pathological thrombopoiesis. Cancer Chemother Pharmacol 1996;38S:S99-S102.
3. Galmiche MC, Vogel CA, Delaloye AB, et al. Combined effects on interleukin-3 and interleukin-11 on hematopoiesis in irradiated mice. Exp Hematol 1996;24:1298-306.
4. Redlich CA, Gao X, Rockwell S, Kelly M, Elias JA. IL-11 enhances survival and decreases TNF production after radiation-induced thoracic injury. J Immunol 1996;157:1705-10.

Interleukin 12

Vellalore N. Kakanaiah, Ph.D.

Interleukin 12, originally known as the natural killer cell stimulatory factor, is a multifunctional cytokine produced by monocytes/macrophages, B cells, and other accessory cells in response to bacteria, bacterial products, or parasites.[1] IL-12 induces IFN-γ secretion by T and NK cells, acts as a growth factor for activated T and NK cells, enhances the lytic activity of NK/lymphokine-activated killer (NK/LAK) cells, and facilitates specific cytotoxic T-cell (CTL) responses.[2,3] IL-12 plays an important role in stimulating the differentiation of T-helper type 1 (Th1) responses from naive Th cells by acting as a co-stimulus required for maximum IFN-γ secretion by antigen-activated Th1 cells.[4] IL-12 indirectly stimulates B-cell growth and switching of IgG alloantibody subclass through the production of IFN-γ.[5,6] IL-12 induces effective anti-tumor immunity along with other co-stimuli such as IL-2 or B7.1 of HIV.[7,8] IL-12 production is decreased in cells from HIV-positive individuals.[9] In cultures, gp120 of HIV is an inducer of IL-12 expression in monocytes/macrophages and is dependent on IFN-γ.[10] IL-12 is capable of indirectly down-regulating HIV proliferation in macrophage cultures reconstituted with autologous PBMC and of directly suppressing HIV replication in purified macrophage cultures.[11] IL-12 restores IFN-γ production and cytotoxic responses in visceral leishmaniasis,[12] and inhibits endotoxin-induced inflammation in the eye.[13]

REFERENCES
1. Wolf SF, Sieburth D, Sypek J. Interleukin 12: a key modulator of immune function. Stem Cells 1994;12:154-68.
2. Trinchieri G. Interleukin-12: a cytokine produced by antigen-presenting cells with immunoregulatory functions in the generation of T-helper cells type 1 and cytotoxic lymphocytes. Blood 1994;84:4008-27.
3. Hendrzak JA, Brunda MJ. Interleukin-12: biologic activity, therapeutic utility, and role in disease. Lab Invest 1995;72:619-37.

4. Murphy EE, Terres G, Macatonia SE, et al. B7 and interleukin 12 cooperates for proliferation and interferon-γ production by mouse T helper clones that are unresponsive to B7 costimulation. J Exp Med 1994;180:223-31.

5. Li L, Young D, Wolf SF, Choi YS. Interleukin-12 stimulates B cell growth by inducing IFN-γ. Cell Immunol 1996;168:133-40.

6. Gracie JA, Bradley JA. Interleukin-12 induces interferon-γ-dependent switching of IgG alloantibody subclass. Eur J Immunol 1996;26:1217-21.

7. Wigginton JM, Kuhns DB, Back TC, Brunda MJ, Wiltrout RH, Cox GW. Interleukin 12 primes macrophages for nitric oxide production *in vivo* and restores depressed nitric oxide production by macrophages from tumor-bearing mice: implications for the antitumor activity of interleukin 12 and/or interleukin 2. Cancer Res 1996;56:1131-6.

8. Zitvogel L, Robbins PD, Storkus WJ, et al. Interleukin-12 and B7.1 co-stimulation cooperate in the production of effective antitumor immunity and therapy of established tumors. Eur J Immunol 1996;26:1335-41.

9. Chougnet C, Wynn TA, Clerici M, et al. Molecular analysis of decreased interleukin-12 production in persons infected with human immunodeficiency virus. J Infec Dis 1996;176:46-53.

10. Fantuzzi L, Gessani S, Borghi P, et al. Induction of interleukin-12 (IL-12) by recombinant glycoprotein gp120 of human immunodeficiency virus type 1 in human monocytes/macrophages: requirement of gamma interferon for IL-12 secretion. J Virol 1996;70:4121-4.

11. Akridge R, Reed SG. Interleukin-12 decreases human immunodeficiency virus type 1 replication in human macrophage cultures reconstituted with autologous peripheral blood mononuclear cells. J Infect Dis 1996;173:559-64.

12. Bacellar O, Brodskyn C, Guerreiro J, et al. Interleukin-12 restores interferon-γ production and cytotoxic responses in visceral leishmaniasis. J Infect Dis 1996;173:1515-8.

13. Whitcup SM, Rizzo LV, Lai JC, Hayashi S, Gazzinelli R, Chan C-C. IL-12 inhibits endotoxin-induced inflammation in the eye. Eur J Immunol 1996;26:995-9.

Leukotrienes

Jeffrey W. Terryberry, B.S.

Leukotrienes are unsaturated eicosanoids produced from the phospholipid derivative, arachidonic acid (AA). 5-lipoxygenase (5-LO) produces LTA_4 and 5-hydroperoxyeicosatetraenoic acid in the AA cascade, and its activity is stimulated by 5-LO activating protein (FLAP) as well as by receptor-mediated activation, immune complex formation, tissue trauma, glucocorticoids, cytokines, growth factors, neurotransmitters and neuropeptides.[1] LTB_4 is produced from LTA_4 by a hydrolase; whereas, conjugation of LTA_4 to glutathione by LTC_4 synthetase yields LTC_4. LTC_4 is converted to LTD_4 and LTE_4 by γ-glutamyl transpeptidase and dipeptidase. N-acetylation, oxidations, and peroxidations yield a variety of other mediating metabolites.[1,2] Neutrophils acting in the first line of natural nonspecific defense, are stimulated by LTB_4 to adhere to epithelium, degranulate, express C3b receptors and produce superoxide with enhanced cytotoxicity.

Neutrophil chemotactic and chemokinetic activity is often used as a bioassay for LTB_4 measurement. LTB_4 also induces macrophage cytokine production and phagocytosis, natural killer cell cytotoxic activity, $CD8^+$ T killer activity, B cell Ig production, mucous secretion and the release of more AA. LTC_4 and LTD_4 also prime macrophages to secrete cytokines as well as modulate glutathione antioxidant potential, enhance eosinophil motility, natural killer cell cytotoxicity, and induce fibroblasts to produce collagen.[1]

LT antagonists and LO inhibitors such as methotrexate, colchicine, NHGA, BAY-x-7195, loratadine and SB20947 function as immunosuppressors and are emerging as important therapeutic agents.[1,3-6] LTE_3 and LTE_4 correlate with chronic inflammation; elevated urinary LTE_4 is seen in obstructive jaundice, malnutrition, liver cirrhosis, hepatorenal syndrome, SLE and cystic fibrosis.[1,7-10] LTB_4 is upregulated in HIV infection and in acute and chronic respiratory diseases, including asthma, rheumatoid arthritis, psoriasis, neoplasia, rhinitis, inflammatory bowel disease, ischemia and tissue transplantation. LTC_4 and LTD_4 are elevated in bronchoalveolar lavage fluid of asthmatic patients and in nasal discharge of rhinitis patients. Plasma levels of LTB$_4$ and LTE$_4$ are also increased in pulmonary diseases. Plasma LTC$_4$ concentrations are elevated in Kawasaki disease.[1,6,11-17]

REFERENCES

1. Denzlinger C. Biology and pathophysiology of leukotrienes. Crit Rev Oncol Hematol 1996;23:167-223.
2. Devchand PR, Keller H, Peters JM, Vazquez M, Gonzales FJ, Wahli W. The PPARα-leukotriene B$_4$ pathway to inflammation control. Nature 1996;384:39-43.
3. Sarau HM, Foley JJ, Schmidt DB, et al. SB 209247, a high affinity LTB$_4$ receptor antagonist demonstating potent antiinflammatory activity. Adv Prostaglandin Thromboxane Leukot Res 1995;23:275-7.
4. Tasaka K, Kamei C, Akagi M, et al. Effect of loratadine on immediate and delayed type hypersensitivity reactions. Arzneimittelforschung 1995;45:796-804.
5. Tanaka H, Nagai H, Takeda H, Yamaguchi S, Matsuo A, Inagaki N. Prostaglandins 1995;50:269-85.
6. Smith LJ. Leukotrienes in asthma. The potential therapeutic role of antileukotriene agents. Arch Intern Med 1996;156:2181-9.
7. Greally P, Cook AJ, Sampson AP, et al. Atopic children with cystic fibrosis have increased urinary leukotriene E4 concentrations and more severe pulmonary disease. J Allergy Clin Immunol 1994;93:100-7.
8. Hackshaw KV, Voelkel NL, Thomas RB, Westcott JY. Urine leukotriene E4 levels are elevated in patients with active systemic lupus erythematosus. J Rheumatol 1992;19:252-8.
9. Mayatepek K, Pecher G. Increased excretion of endogenous urinary leukotriene E4 in extrahepatic cholestasis. Clin Chim Acta 1993;218:185-92.
10. Uemura M, Buchholz U, Kojima H, et al. Cysteinyl leukotrienes in the urine of patients with liver disease. Hepatology 1994;20:804-12.
11. Lipschik GY, Doerfler ME, Kovacs JA, et al. Leukotriene B4 and interleukin-8 in human immunodeficiency virus-related pulmonary disease. Chest 1993;104:763-9.
12. Crea AEG, Nakhosteen JA, Lee TH. Mediator concentrations in bronchoalveolar lavage fluid of patients with mild asymptomatic bronchial asthma. Eur Respir J 1992;5:190-5.
13. Seggev JS, Thornton WH, Edes TE. Serum leukotriene B4 levels in patients with obstructive pulmonary disease. Chest 1991;99:289-91.
14. Shindo K, Miyakawa K, Fukumura M. Plasma levels of leukotriene B4 in asthmatic patients. Int J Tissue React 1993;15:181-4.
15. Wenzel SE, Larsen GL, Johnston K, et al. Elevated levels of leukotriene C$_4$ in bronchoalveolar lavage fluid from atopic asthmatics after endobronchial allergen challenge. Am Rev Respir Dis 1990;141:1453-8.
16. Kohi F, Miyagawa H, Agrawal DK, et al. Generation of leukotriene B$_4$ and C$_4$ from granulocytes of normal controls, allergic rhinitis, and asthmatic subjects. Ann Allergy 1990;65:228-32.
17. Sasai K, Fukuda Y, Furukawa S, Yabuta K. Plasma immunoreactive leukotriene C$_4$ levels in patients with Kawasaki disease. Ann Allergy 1990;65:477-80.

Platelet-Activating Factor

Alaa E. Ahmed, Ph.D.

Platelet-activating factor (PAF) (1-*O*-alkyl-2-acetyl-*sn*-glycero-3 phosphocholine) belongs to a family of acetylated glycerophospholipids and is synthesized via the remodeling pathway (acelation of lyso PAF by the enzyme acetyltransferase) or by the '*de novo* pathway' through the action of the enzyme cholinphosphotransferase on ether linked phospholipid.[1] PAF is produced by a variety of inflammatory cells including platelets, neutrophils, alveolar macrophages, eosinophils and vascular endothelial cells.[2] In man, mast cells synthesize, but do not release PAF.[1] PAF is thought to be involved in a variety of pathophysiologic conditions including arterial thrombosis, acute inflammation, endotoxic shock, acute allergic diseases and gastrointestinal ulceration.[1,3]

PAF is released in increased quantities in the sputum of patients with asthma and chronic lung disease, in nasal secretions and skin after antigen challenge, and in blood after cold challenge in cold-induced urticaria. Inhalation of PAF causes transient bronchospasm, eosinophil influx and increased microvascular permeability in the central and peripheral airways. Intradermal injection of PAF causes wheal and flare followed by an indurated red papule.[3,4] Severe childhood asthma is associated with deficiency of specific hydrolases which metabolize PAF.[4] Deficiency of PAF acetylhydrolase is an autosomal recessive condition associated with severe asthma in children.[5] Leucocytes express high and low affinity PAF receptors in addition to intracellular PAF receptors.[6] PAF is postulated to mediate normal responses including reproduction, hemostasis and memory.[7] Several synthetic PAF antagonists subjected to long-term clinical studies are not promising for asthma treatment.[3]

REFERENCES
1. Minhas BS, Ripps BA, Zhu YP, et al. Platelet activating factor and conception. Am J Rep Immunol 1996;35:267-71.
2. Lopez-Novoa LM, Rodriguez-Barbero A, Eleno N. The role of platelet-activating factor and the effect of PAF blocking receptors on the outcome of ARF. Renal Failure 1996;18:489-99.
3. Kuitert L, Barnes NC. PAF and asthma: time for an appraisal. Clin Exp Allergy 1995;25:1159-62.
4. Chung KF. Platelet-activating factor in inflammation and pulmonary disorders. Clin Sci 1992;83:127-38.
5. Stafforni DM, Satoh K, Atkinson DL, et al. Platelet activating factor acetylhydrolase deficiency: a missense mutation near the active site on an anti-inflammatory phospholipase. J Clin Invest 1996;97:2784-91.
6. Svetlov S, Nigam S. Evidence for the presence of specific high affinity cytosolic binding sites for platelet-activating factor in human neutrophils. Biochem Biophys Res Commun 1993;190:162-6.
7. Prescott SM, McIntyre TM, Zimmerman GA, Stafforini DM. Inflammation as an early component of atherosclerosis and vascular damage. A role for P-selectin and platelet-activating factor. Japn Circ J 1996;60:137-41.

Prostaglandins

Jeffrey W. Terryberry, B.S.

The initial inflammatory event in anaphylaxis is mediated by histamine, serotonin, bradykinin and substance P, and is subsequently maintained by eicosanoids, cytokines and growth factors.[1] Inhibition of prostanoid formation using non-steriodal anti-inflammatory drugs like indomethacin and diclofenac, ameliorates the classical signs of inflammation.[1,2] Phospholipid-derived arachidonic acid (C20:4), liberated by phospholipase A2 and D, is the substrate for prostaglandin (PG) synthesis by cyclooxygenase (COX). The COX-2 isozyme is also regulated by glucocorticoids (corticosterone, dexamethasone, prednisone). PLA_2 inhibition blocks the synthesis of PGs.[1,3] IL-1, -2, TNF, PAF, EGF, CSF, PDGF, bFGF and endothelin stimulate COX activity in fibroblasts, synoviocytes, macrophages, neutrophils, endothelial cells, astrocytes and mesengial cells; whereas, IL-10 and TGF are inhibitory.[1,4] PGE_2 formation from PGH results in edema, increased vascular permeability, nociception, esophagitis and erythema; PGI_2 is also vasodilatory; whereas, $PGF_{2\alpha}$ is vasoconstrictive.[1,5,6] However, in chronic inflammation, persistent PGE_2 concentrations are immunosuppressive, causing reductions in T-cell cytokines and B-cell Ig, as well as LTB_4 inhibition, decreased nitric oxide synthesis, reduced atherosclerosis and decreased oxidative burst in neutrophils.[1] The bicyclic prostanoid, prostacyclin, is formed from 6-keto-$PGF_{1\alpha}$ and reduces platelet aggregation. Proinflammatory cytokines 1L-1 and -6 stimulate the production of PGI_2 which is an antithrombogenic inhibitor of platelet aggregation and of PLA_2 activity. $PGF_{2\alpha}$ regulates edema induced by PGE_2 and antagonizes the release of histamine, 5-HT, and tachykinins. Mast cell-derived PGD_2, formed from PGH_2, also inhibits platelet aggregation and causes bronchoconstriction.[1,7] COX inhibition reduces PGE_2 formation in pleural effusions during acute pleurisy, and decreases prothrombotic thromboxane formation in cardiovascular diseases.[1,5] Rheumatoid arthritis synovial fluid contains elevated PGE_2 concentrations.[8] Gastric and renal side effects of aspirin are associated with inhibition of the cytoprotective effects of PGE_1, PGE_2, and PGI_2 against chronic (T-cell-dependent) inflammation. Tumor angiogenesis involves PGE_2 upregulation and can be inhibited by PGH_2 synthase inhibitors.[1,9] The acute inflammatory mediator, nitric oxide (NO) can regulate prostanoid formation, and PGE_2 regulates NO synthase; both NO and its synthase are upregulated in autoimmune diseases.[10-13] Thus, the measurement and quantitation of PGs and other ecosanoids in biological samples is an important issue in studies of inflammation, renal function, cardiovascular disease and cancer.[14] A tandem and electrospray mass spectrometry assay concentration resolve eight eicosanoids with equivalent sensitivity as GC-MS, HPLC, and immunoassays (pg/mL).[14]

REFERENCES

1. Appleton I, Tomlinson A, Willoughby DA. Induction of cyclo-oxygenase and nitric oxide synthase in inflammation. Adv Pharmacol 1996;35:27-78.
2. Tonussi CR, Ferreira SH. Mechanism of diclofenac analgesia: direct blockage of inflammatory sensitization. Eur J Pharmacol 1994;251:173-9.
3. DeWitt DL, Meade EA. Serum and glucocorticoid regulation of gene transcription and expression of the prostaglandin H synthase-1 and prostaglandin H synthase-2 isozymes. Arch Biochem Biophys 1993;306:94-102.
4. Mertz PM, DeWitt DL, Stetler-Stevenson WG, Wahl LM. Interleukin 10 suppression of monocyte prostaglandin H synthase-2. J Biol Chem 1994;269:21322-9.
5. Harada Y, Hatanaka K, Kawamura M, et al. Role of prostaglandin H synthase-2 in prostaglandin E_2 formation in rat carrageenin-induced pleurisy. Prostaglandins 1996;51:19-33.
6. Morgan G. Deleterious effects of prostaglandin E2 in reflux oesophagitis. Med Hypotheses 1996;46:42-4.
7. Bui KC, Hammerman C, Hirschi RB, et al. Plasma prostanoids in neonates with pulmonary hypertension treated with conventional therapy and with extracorporeal membrane oxygenation. J Thorac Cardiovasc Surg 1991;101:973-83.
8. Crofford LJ, Wilder RL, Ristimaki AP, et al. Cyclooxygenase-1 and -2 expression in rheumatoid synovial tissues. Effects of interleukin-1β, phorbol ester and corticosteroids. J Clin Invest 1994;93:1095-1101.
9. Peterson HI. Tumour angiogenesis inhibition by prostaglandin synthetase inhibitors. Anticancer Res 1986;6:251-3.
10. Swierkosz TA, Mitchell JA, Warner TD, Botting RM, Vane JR. Co-induction of nitric oxide synthase and cyclo-oxygenase: interactions between nitric oxide and prostanoids. Br J Pharmacol 1995;114:1335-42.
11. Salvemini D, Seibert K, Masferrer JL, Misko TP, Currie MG, Needleman P. Endogenous nitric oxide enhances prostaglandin production in a model of renal inflammation. J Clin Invest 1994;93:1940-7.
12. Tetsuka T, Daphna-Iken D, Srivastava SK, Baier LD, DuMaine J, Morrison AR. Cross-talk between cycloxygenase and niric oxide pathways: prostaglandin E_2 negatively modulates induction of nitric oxide synthase by interleukin-1. Proc Natl Acad Sci USA 1994;91:12168-72.
13. Weinberg JB, Granger DL, Pisetsky DS, et al. The role of nitric oxide in the pathogenesis of spontaneous murine autoimmune disease: increase niric oxide production and nitric oxide synthase expression in MRL-lpr/lpr mice, and reduction of spontaneous glomerularnephritis and arthritis by orally administered NG-monomethyl-L-arginine. J Exp Med 1994;179:651-60.
14. Margalit A, Duffin KL, Isakson PC. Rapid quantitation of a large scope of eicosanoids in two models of inflammation: development of an electrospray and tandem mass spectrometry method and application to biological studies. Anal Biochem 1996;235:73-81.

Thromboxane A_2

Alaa E. Ahmed, Ph.D.

Thromboxane A_2 (TXA$_2$), the most potent platelet-aggregating agonist and vasoconstrictor isolated to date, is formed from PGG$_2$ and PGH$_2$ (generated by the cyclo-oxygenase pathway) by the enzyme thromboxane synthetase.[1] TXA$_2$ is very unstable (half-life = 30 seconds) and undergoes rapid hydrolysis to its inactive, stable end product TXB$_2$. The major source of TXA$_2$ is platelets, but it can also be generated by monocytes.[2] Platelets are the source of circulating TXA$_2$ involved in blood clotting; neutrophils are the cellular source in inflammation.[1] The principal action of TXA$_2$ in inflammation is to induce platelet aggregation, vasoconstriction, bronchoconstriction and bronchial hyperresponsiveness. TXA$_2$ is also involved in the late allergen-induced cutaneous responses.[2,3] See in this Chapter: **Prostaglandins.**

REFERENCES

1. Appleton I, Tomlinson A, Willoughby DA. Induction of cyclo-oxygenase and nitric oxide synthase in inflammation. Adv Pharmacol. 1996;35:27-77.
2. Ohtsuka T, Matsumaru S, Uchida K, et al. Pathogenic role of thromboxane A2 in immediate food hypersensitivity reactions in children. Ann Allergy Asthma Immunol 1996;77:55-9.
3. Saito M, Fujimura M, Sakamoto S, et al. Involvement of arachidonate cyclo-oxygenase products in bronchial hyperresponsivness induced by subthreshold concetration of aerosolized thromboxane A2 analogue (STA2) in guinea pigs. Allergy 1992;47:181-4.

Chapter 7
Evaluation of Complement

AH50

Alaa E. Ahmed, Ph.D.

The functional activity of the alternative pathway is assessed by evaluating the alternative pathway (AP) hemolytic assay (AH50) using complement-mediated lysis of rabbit erythrocytes in Mg^{2+}-EGTA buffer.[1] EGTA chelates Ca^{2+} required for the assembly of the C1 macromolecule of complement, thereby inhibiting activity of the classical pathway.[1,2]

The AH50 assay is a useful screening tool for homozygous deficiencies of AP components including C3, factor I, factor B, properdin, factor H and factor D.[2] Deficiencies of factor I or H, which are fluid-phase regulatory proteins of the AP, causes secondary deficiency of C3, properdin and factor B due to uncontrolled consumption of those proteins.[2,3] Absence of hemolysis in both the AH50 and CH50 assays is a strong indication for deficiency in one of the complement terminal pathway components (C5 to C9). Normal AH50 values and absence of lysis in CH50 indicates a classical pathway component deficiency (C1, C2, or C4). Normal CH50 and absence of hemolysis in AH50 is a strong indication for AP component deficiency.[2,3] Absence of lysis strongly suggests homozygous deficiency; whereas, low levels of lysis in AH50 or CH50 assay is evidence for either heterozygous deficiency or complement activation.[2] Hemolytic functional assays for individual complement components are useful for defining homozygous and to some extent heterozygous deficiencies, as well as mutations that produce functionally inactive complement proteins, for which deficiencies cannot be defined by quantitation alone.[2,4] In general, AP deficiency is usually associated with recurrent bacterial infections.[2] To date, factor B deficiency is not reported.[2] Homozygous deficiency of factor H is associated with glomerulonephritis, recurrent pyogenic infection, hemolytic-uremic syndrome, systemic lupus erythematosus or good health.[2,5] Deficiency of factor D is associated with recurrent upper respiratory tract infection (*Neisseria* spp.).[2] The kidneys play a major role in clearance and catabolism of factor D, which is filtered by the glomeruli and catabolized in the proximal tubular epithelium.[2] EIAs for quantitation of components of the alternative pathway are promising but their clinical utility is not established.[6] See in this Chapter: **CH50** and **Complement Split Products** as well as Chapter 6: **C3a, C4a and C5a Anaphylatoxins**.

REFERENCES
1. Servais G, Walmagh J, Duchateau J. Simple quantitative haemolytic microassay for determination of complement alternative pathway activation (AP50). J Immunol Methods 1991;140:93-100.
2. Ahmed AEE, Peter JB. Clinical utility of complement assessment [Minireview]. Clin Diagn Lab Immunol 1995;2:507-17.
3. Walport MJ, Lachmann PJ. Complement deficiencies and abnormalities of the complement system in lupus erythematosus and related disorders. Curr Opin Rheumatol 1990;2:661-3.
4. Whaley K. Measurement of complement. In: Whaley K, editor. Methods in Complement for the Clinical Immunologists. Edinburgh: Churchill Livingston, Ltd., 985:77-139.
5. Walport MJ. Complement deficiency and disease. Br J Rheumatol 1993;32:269-73.
6. Oppermann M, Baumgaten H, Brandt E, Gottsleben W, Kurts C, Gotze O. Quantitation of the alternative pathway of complement (APC) by enzyme-linked immunosorbent assays. J Immunol Methods 1990;133:181-90.

C1 Inhibitor Deficiency and Angioedema

Alaa E. Ahmed, Ph.D.

Human C1 Inhibitor (C1 INH), a serine protease inhibitor with a molecular weight of 105 kd that belongs to the serpin family,[1] is a major inhibitor of the inflammatory response via its inactivation of the C1r and C1s proteases of the complement system, factors XIa and XIIa of the coagulation system, plasmin of the fibrinolytic system and kallikrein of the kinin system.[1,2] Hereditary or acquired deficiency of C1 INH causes angioedema in skin or mucosa of the extremities, face, gastrointestinal tract and upper airways.[3] Type I and II hereditary angioedema (HAE) are autosomal dominant disorders. Type I HAE (~85% of kindreds) is characterized by low plasma levels of C1 INH protein and decreased C1 INH functional activity associated with partial deletions and/or duplications of the C1 INH gene on chromosome 11); the remaining C1 INH is apparently normal, catalytically active and present at 5-30% of reference range concentrations. In type II HAE (~15% of kindreds), normal to elevated levels of C1 INH protein are consistent with structural gene defects manifest by the presence of both a dysfunctional mutant protein and <50% of the normal protein.[4] Decreased synthesis of normal C1 INH (as expected in heterozygotes for types I and II HAE) is accompanied by elevated fractional catabolic rates for normal C1 INH so that serum concentrations of normal C1 INH are reduced to <50% of the usual reference range.[2,3]

The most common variety of acquired deficiency of C1 INH[4] (due to increased consumption as opposed to the decreased synthesis and increased consumption in HAE) is type I, which is associated with benign or malignant B-cell lymphoproliferative disorders.[5] A less common form (type II) is associated with autoantibodies to C1 INH,[6,7] including one variety in which the autoantibody facilitates proteolytic cleavage of normal C1 INH to an inactive, structurally modified protein with a molecular weight of 96 kd.[3] The decreases in serum C1q protein in the acquired forms of angioedema distinguish them from HAE. All forms of HAE and acquired deficiency of C1 INH respond to attenuated androgens, but individuals with acquired deficiency require higher doses. Angiotensin converting enzyme inhibitors can precipitate angioedema in patients with a history of idiopathic angioedema.[8]

REFERENCES
1. Nielsen EW, Gran JT, Straume B, et al. Hereditary angio-oedema: new clinical observations and autoimmune screening, complement and kallikrein-kinin analyses. J Intern Med 1996;239:119-30.
2. Shoemaker LR, Schurman SJ, Donaldson VH, Davis AE III. Hereditary angioneurotic oedema: characterization of plasma kinin and vascular permeability-enhancing activities. Clin Exp Immunol 1994;95:22-8.
3. Davis AE III, Cicardi M. C1 inhibitor autoantibodies. In: Peter JB, Shoenfeld Y, editors. Autoantibodies. Amsterdam: Elsevier Science B.V., 1996:126-31.
4. Winsieski JJ, Knauss TC, Yike I, et al. Unique C1 inhibitor in a kindered without angioedema: I. A mutant C1 inhibitor that inhibits C1s but not C1r. J Immunol 1994;152:3199-3209.
5. Chevailler A, Arlaud G, Ponard D, et al. C1 inhibitor binding monoclonal immunoglobulins in three patients with acquired angioneurotic edema. J Allergy Clin Immunol 1996;97:998-1008.
6. Mandle R, Baron C, Roux E, et al. Acquired C1 inhibitor deficiency as a result of an autoantibody to the reactive region of C1 inhibitor. J Immunol 1994;152:4680-5.
7. He S, Tsang S, North J, et al. Epitope mapping of C1 inhibitor autoantibodies from patients with acquired C1 inhibitor deficiency. J Immunol 1996;156:2009-13.
8. Acker CG, Greenberg A. Angioedema induced by the angiotensin II blocker Losartan [Letter]. N Engl J Med 1995;333:1572.

C1q Autoantibodies

Alaa E. Ahmed, Ph.D.

C1q, the 410 kd glycoprotein recognition unit of the C1 macromolecule of complement,[1] binds to the Fc domain of immunoglobulins in CIC and initiates the activation of the classical complement pathway.[1] Autoantibodies to the C1q molecule are present in SLE patients (14-52%), hypocomplementemic urticarial vasculitis syndrome (HUVS) (100%), RA (5% in uncomplicted RA and 77% of patients with RA complicated with Felty syndrome), MPGN type 1 (73%), MPGN type II and III (45%), mixed connective tissue disease (94%) and polyarterities nodosa (42%).[1,2] The IgG isotype, which is more common than IgA or IgM, is generally found in lupus nephritis.[2,3] Increasing levels of C1q autoantibodies predict renal flares in SLE patients (71% sensitivity, 92% specificity, positive predictive value 50% and negative predictive value 97%).[1,4]

HUVS, a relatively rare condition which can coexist with SLE,[3] is characterized by reduced serum C1q and recurrent idiopathic urticaria with leukocytoclastic vasculitis. High frequencies of angioedema, ocular inflammation, glomerulonephritis, uvetis, arthritis, arthralgia, neurologic abnormalities and obstructive plumonary disease are common findings in HUVS.[3] HUVS' relationship to SLE is uncertain, but the general absence of autoantibodies, and in particular, the absence of dsDNA autoantibodies, suggests that HUVS is not a subset of SLE.[5]

REFERENCES
1. Wener MH, Mannik M. C1q antibodies. In: Peter JB, Shoenfeld Y, editors. Autoantibodies. Amsterdam: Elsevier Science B.V., 1996:132-8.
2. D'Cruz DP, Wisnieski JJ, Asherson RA, Khamashta MA, Hughes GRV. Autoantibodies in systemic lupus erythematosus and urticarial vasculitis. J Rheumatol 1995;22:1669-73.
3. Winsnieski JJ, Baer AN, Christensen J, et al. Hypocomplementemic urticarial vasculitis syndrome. Clinical and serologic findings in 18 patients. Medicine 1995;74:24-41.
4. Coremans IEM, Spronk PE, Bootsma H, et al. Changes in antibodies to C1q predict renal relapses in systemic lupus erythematosus. Am J Kidney Dis 1995;26:595-601.
5. Wisnieski LL, Jones S. Comparison of autoantibodies to the collagen-like region of C1q in hypocomplementemic urticarial vasculitis syndrome and systemic lupus erythematosus. J Immunol 1992;148:1396-1403.

CH50

Alaa E. Ahmed, Ph.D.

Total complement hemolytic activity of the classical pathway and terminal sequence of complement activation is measured by the CH50 assay, with results expressed in hemolytic units which represent the amount of serum required to lyse 50% of sheep red cells sensitized with rabbit IgG antibody (hemolysin).[1,2] A normal CH50 assay indicates that C1 through C9 are present in the serum being tested. However, even in the presence of a normal CH50, the absolute concentrations of some complement components (e.g., C3 or C4) can be significantly lower than normal, because normal serum contains C3 and C4 in substantial excess of that required to yield a normal CH50 result.[2,3] CH50 can be used to assess integrity of both the classical and terminal sequence of complement activation, but cannot be used as a sensitive test for *in vivo* complement activation.[2,4] In general, no lysis in the CH50 assay suggests a homozygous deficiency in one of the classical or terminal complement proteins (C1 to C9). Low levels of CH50 suggests either a heterozygous deficiency or high complement turn-over.[2]

During pregnancy, the ratio of CH50 to Ba concentration is higher in patients with preeclampsia than in those with active SLE. A decline in the C3 or C4 concentration or CH50, accompanied by elevation in C4d, Ba and SC5b-9 concentrations, differentiates a lupus flare from non-SLE complication of pregnancy.[2] The classical method for CH50 determination is the hemolytic assay, which offers higher sensitivity than other methodologies.[2] See in this Chapter: **AH50, Complement Components** and **Complement Split Products** as well as Chapter 6: **C3a, C4a and C5a Anaphylatoxins.**

REFERENCES
1. Abbal M, Tkaczuk J, Praud C, Msayeh F, Ohayon E. Computer-assisted kinetic assay for quantitation of total complement activity. Complement Inflamm 1991;8:92-103.
2. Ahmed AEE, Peter JB. Clinical utility of complement assessment. Clin Diagn Lab Immunol 1995;2:509-17.
3. Hebert LA, Cosio FG, Neff JC. Diagnostic significance of hypocomplementemia. Kidney Int 1991;39:811-21.
4. Whaley K. The complement system. In: Whaley K, Loos M, Weiler JM, editors. Complement in health and disease. Boston: Kluwer Academic Publishers, 1993:1-32.

Complement Components

Alaa E. Ahmed, Ph.D.

Homozygous deficiencies of complement classical pathway components (C1, C2 and C4) are largely associated with SLE or SLE-like disease;[1,2] whereas, deficiencies of the alternative pathway components (factor H, factor I, factor D, properdin) and the terminal sequence of complement are associated with recurrent infections and pyogenic infections.[3,4] Many data indicate that serum C3 concentrations are likely to change from normal to abnormal as SLE changes from quiescent to active.[5] Three distinctive patterns of terminal complement component deficiencies are seen in idiopathic membranoproliferative glomerulonephritis (MPGN) and acute post-infectious glomerulonephritis: depression of all the terminal pathway components (C5-C9) as well as C3 is seen in patients with MPGN types I and III[6] and is associated with a corresponding increase in C3-properdin dependent nephritic factor (C3Nef);[7] C3 and C5 decreased but C6-C9 usually within the normal range in APGN;[5] and C5-C9 normal but C3 decreased in MPGN type II.[6] See in this Chapter: **AH50** and **CH50**.

REFERENCES

1. Colten HR. Complement deficiencies. Annu Rev Immunol 1992;10:809-34.
2. Lachmann PJ. Complement deficiency and the pathogenesis of autoimmune immune complex disease. Chem Immunol 1990;49:245-63.
3. Densen P. Infectious consequences of complement deficiency states. Clinical Immunology Newsletter 1991;11:1-10.
4. Ahmed AEE, Peter JB. Clinical utility of complement assessment. Clin Diagn Lab Immunol 1995;2:507-17.
5. Hebert LA, Cosio FG, Neff JC. Diagnostic significance of hypocomplementemia. Kidney Int 1991;39:811-21.
6. Clardy CW, Forristal J, Strife CF, West CD. Serum terminal complement component levels in hypocomplementemic glomerulonephritidis. Clin Immunol Immunopathol 1989;50:307-20.
7. Tanuma Y, Ohi H, Hatano M. Two types of C3 nephritic factor: properdin C3Nef and properdin-independent C3Nef. Clin Immunol Immunopathol 1990;56:226-38.

Complement Receptors

Alaa E. Ahmed, Ph.D.

Regulation of complement activation is largely mediated by a group of proteins encoded as a cluster of genes on chromosome 1 known as regulators of complement gene family (RCA).[1] The RCA proteins are C3b and/or C4b binding proteins that regulate complement activation either by accelerating the decay of complement convertases or by acting as co-factors for Factor I-mediated cleavage of C3b and C4b.[2] Factor H and C4 binding protein (C4BP) are fluid-phase RCA proteins; whereas, decay accelerating factor (DAF), membrane co-factor (MCP), complement receptor 1 (CR1), and complement receptor 2 (CR2) are membrane-bound RCA proteins. Clearance of CIC is mediated in part by CR1 expressed on erythrocytes as well as CR3 and CR4 expressed on RES cells.[2,3] Erythrocyte CR1 is reduced in 66% of patients with SLE,[2] as well as autoimmune hemoloytic anemia, paroxysmal nocturnal hemoglobinuria, AIDS and lepromatous leprosy.[2,4]

Lower CR1 expression is not genetically linked with SLE but is acquired.[2] Normal B cells (expressing CR2) are capable of activating the complement alternative pathway in a CR2-dependent fashion.[5] There is an inverse relationship between SLE disease activity index and the expression of CR2 on SLE B cells.[5] Recombinant soluble CR1 blocks complement activation in human serum.[2] Flow cytometric assays are available to measure and define the cellular expression and deficiencies of complement receptors and membrane regulatory proteins.[4]

REFERENCES

1. Hourcade D, Garcia AD, Post TW, et al. Analysis of the human regulators of complement activation (RCA) gene cluster with yeast artificial chromosomes (YACs). Genomics 1992;12:289-300.
2. Birmingham DJ. Erythrocyte complement receptors. Crit Rev Immunol 1995;15:133-54.
3. Witte T, Dumoulin F-L, Gessner JE, et al. Defect of a complement receptor 3 epitope in a patient with systemic lupus erythematosus. J Clin Invest 1993,92:1181-7.
4. Ahmed AEE, Peter JB. Clinical utility of complement assessment. Clin Diagn Lab Immunol 1995;2:507-17.

5. Marquart HV, Svendsen A, Rasmussen JM, et al. Complement receptor expression and activation of complement cascade on B lymphocytes from patients with systemic lupus erythematosus (SLE). Clin Exp Immunol 1995;101:60-5.

Complement Split Products

Alaa E. Ahmed, Ph.D.

Complement activation can be evaluated indirectly by quantitation of native complement components (e.g., C3, C4 and factor B) or complement functional assays (e.g., CH50 and AH50), which have limited utility, or directly by quantitation of complement activation products, which is more sensitive and reliable.[1,2] Complement split products are classified as anaphylatoxins (C3a, C4a and C5a), complement activation fragments (C4d, C3b, iC3b, C3d, C3c, Ba, Bb) and multimolecular complexes (C1r:C1s:C1 inhibitor, C3b:Bb:Properdin and SC5b-9).[1,2]

iC3b and C3d concentrations are a marker of disease activity in SLE. The C3d:total C3 activation index is a better marker of disease severity than C3d alone; C3d is as reliable as C-reactive protein in the diagnosis of neonatal bacterial infection.[3-5] C3d concentrations are elevated in sepsis, renal diseases, atherosclerosis and thermal injury.[2]

Ba, Bb, and C4d concentrations are sensitive markers for SLE and RA disease activity.[2] Concentrations of the multimolecular complexes C1r:C1s:C1 inhibitor, C3b:Bb:Properdin, and SC5b-9 are elevated in SLE, rheumatoid arthritis, leukocytoclastic cutaneous vasculitis, Kawasaki syndrome and acute renal transplant rejection patients.[2] See in this Chapter: **Complement Components**.

REFERENCES
1. Porcel JM, Peahman M, Ensaldi G, Vergani D. Methods for assessing complement activation in the clinical immunology laboratory. J Immunol Methods. 1993;157:1-9.
2. Ahmed AEE, Peter JB. Clinical utility of complement assessment. Clin Diagn Lab Immunol 1995;2:509-17.
3. Rother E, Lang B, Coldway R, Hartung K, Peter HH. Complement split-product C3d as an indicator of disease activity in systemic lupus erythematosus. Clin Rheumatol 1993;12:31-5.
4. Negoro N, Okamura M, Takeda T, et al. The clinical significance of iC3b neoantigen expression in plasma from patients with systemic lupus erythematosus. Arthritis Rheum 1989;32:1233-42.
5. Guillois, Donnou MD, Sizun J, Bendoud B, Youinou P. Comparative study of four tests of bacterial infection in the neonate. Biol Neonate 1994;66:175-81.

Hypocomplementemic Urticaria Vasculitis Syndrome: See in this Chapter: C1q Autoantibodies.

Chapter 8
Viral Infections Associated with Allergy, Asthma and Immunodeficiency States

Epstein-Barr Virus

Madhumita Patnaik, M.D.

Epstein-Barr virus (EBV), a human herpesvirus known to cause infectious mononucleosis, also almost certainly plays a role in the etiology of some carcinomas (nasopharyngeal),[1] lymphomas (Burkitt lymphoma)[2,3] and lymphoproliferative disorders in the presence of immunosuppression.[4,5] Recently, a severe chronic active EBV infection syndrome has been described in which lymphoproliferation continues unabated.[6] Less certain is the etiologic role of EBV in rheumatoid arthritis,[7] Hodgkin disease[8,9] and chronic fatigue syndrome.[10] EBV, especially B-type, was suggested as a cofactor in AIDS, but the relationship of HIV and EBV is still a matter of conjecture.[11] In the persistent generalized lymphadenopathy syndrome and polyclonal B cell activation typical of HIV, EBV plays no direct role.[12] Primary EBV infection in childhood is usually asymptomatic; in adolescents and adults, acute EBV infection results in infectious mononucleosis.[8,13] It is possible that latent and infectious forms of EBV can coexist throughout life in an individual.[13]

The most common test for EBV infection is the rapid slide test (monospot) for heterophile antibody agglutination; the heterophile antibody response is detectable at some point during infectious mononucleosis in ~95% of non-Oriental adolescents and adults and can be detected for several months after acute infection in some individuals.[14,15] Heterophile antibody agglutination is not, however, specific for EBV and is not useful for evaluating chronic disease.[15] EIA is the method of choice; deficiencies including low accuracy, CV $\geq 50\%$, discontinuous readout, and discordance among laboratories are prevalent in titration assays. An EIA using a synthetic EBV nuclear antigen demonstrates IgM antibodies as early as 3-6 days after symptoms appear and can detect antibody response in both heterophile-positive and -negative sera.[16]

Rapid EIA is less reliable and has significant numbers of false-positive results.[17] In the acute phase of infectious mononucleosis, IgM and then IgG antibodies to EBV early antigens (EA), viral capsid antigens (VCA) and nuclear antigens (EBNA) appear in sequence.[14] Thus, either the presence of IgM VCA antibodies or IgM/IgG EA with low or absent EBNA antibodies is indicative of current or recent infection.[18] Combined with positive VCA findings, an IgG to IgM ratio of < 1 by ACIF or EIA can provide diagnostic surety in problem cases.[19] Assaying for avidity of EBV VCA IgG antibodies is also helpful in distinguishing patients with reactivation or latent infection from recent infection.[20]

Persistence of EA and IgG VCA in high titer are indicative of chronic EBV infection.[21] Abnormalities of EBV serology in chronic fatigue patients have not proved clinically useful.[22] DNA hybridization studies not only detect EBV DNA but also help to distinguish between latent (circular, episomal) and replicative (linear) forms in tissue biopsies[23] and whole blood[24] from patients with lymphoproliferative diseases. In patients receiving prophylactic immunoglobulins, serodiagnosis for EBV infection is often problematic; *in situ* hybridization and PCR using peripheral blood mononuclear cells can be used for early and accurate diagnosis of EBV infection in highly vulnerable patients presenting with lymphoproliferative disease.[25] Replicative EBV responds to acyclovir and ganciclovir, and latent EBV does not. PCR can detect EBV genomes in archival tissue[26] and in peripheral blood mononuclear cells of some patients, but detection is not sufficient to ascribe an EBV etiology to symptoms.[27] PCR is useful in detection of EBV in neck metastases, wherein undifferentiated nasopharyngeal carcinoma can be distinguished by the presence of EBV;[28,29] PCR is also valuable as a highly sensitive saliva test for EBV in patients with lymphoproliferative diseases.[30] The association of EBV DNA with patterns of chromosome breakpoint locations in endemic and sporadic Burkitt lymphoma is currently under investigation.[3] Reliable methods for detection and quantitation of EBV RNA are very useful.[31]

REFERENCES

1. Littler E, Baylis SA, Zeng Y, Conway MJ, Mackett M, Arrand JR. Diagnosis of nasopharyngeal carcinoma by means of recombinant Epstein-Barr virus proteins. Lancet 1991;337:685-9.
2. Weiss LM, Movahed LA, Warnke RA, Sklar J. Detection of Epstein-Barr viral genomes in Reed-Sternberg cells of Hodgkin' disease. N Engl J Med 1989;320:502-6.
3. Shiramizu B, Barriga F, Neequaye J, et al. Pattern of chromosomal breakpoint locations in Burkitt's lymphoma: relevance to georgraphy and Epstein-Barr virus association. Blood 1991;77:1516-26.
4. Telenti A, Marshall WF, Smith TF. Detection of Epstein-Barr virus by polymerase chain reaction. J Clin Microbiol 1990;28:2187-90.
5. List AF, Greer JP, Cousar JP, et al. Primary brain lymphoma in the immunocompetent host: relation to Epstein-Barr virus. Mod Pathol 1990;3:609-12.
6. Okano M, Matsumoto S, Osato T, Sakiyama, Thiele GM, Purtilo DT. Severe chronic active Epstein-Barr virus infection syndrome. Clin Microbiol Rev 1991;4:129-35.
7. Lidyard PM, Irving WL. Is there a role for Epstein-Barr virus in the aetiology of rheumatoid arthritis? Br J Rheumatol 1988;27(Suppl II):120-7.
8. Weiss LM, Movahed LA, Warnke RA, Sklar J. Detection of Epstein-Barr viral genomes in Reed-Sternberg cells of Hodgkin's disease. N Engl J Med 1989;1:502-6
9. Samoszuk MK. Epstein-Barr virus in Hodgkin's disease. West J Med 1991;154:92.
10. Hermann Jr WJ. The Epstein-Barr virus and chronic fatigue syndrome [Letter]. JAMA 1989;261:1277-8.
11. Sculley TB, Apolloni A, Hurren L, Moss DJ, Cooper DA. Coinfection with A- and B-type Epstein-Barr virus in human immunodeficiency virus-positive subjects. J Infect Dis 1990;162:643-8.
12. Boyle MJ, Sculley TB, Cooper DA, Turner JJ, Penny R, Sewell WA. Epstein-Barr virus and HIV play no direct role in persistent generalized lymphadenopathy syndrome. Clin Exp Immunol 1992;87:357-61.
13. Niedobitek G, Young LS. Epstein-Barr virus persistence and virus-associated tumors. Lancet 1994;343:333-4.
14. Sumaya CV. Epstein-Barr virus and infectious mononucleosis: a review. J Clin Immunoassay 1989;12:168-74.
15. Merlin TL. Chronic mononucleosis: pitfalls in the laboratory diagnosis. Human Pathol 1986;17:2-8.
16. Smith RS, Rhodes G, Vaughan JH, Horwitz CA, Geltosky JE, Whalley AS. A synthetic peptide for detecting antibodies to Epstein-Barr virus nuclear antigen in sera from patients with infectious mononucleosis. J Infect Dis 1986;154:885-9.
17. Matheson BA, Chisholm SM, Ho-Yen DO. Assessment of rapid ELISA test for detection of Epstein-Barr virus infection. J Clin Pathol 1990;43:691-3.
18. Ho DWT, Field PR, Cunningham AL. Rapid diagnosis of acute Epstein-Barr virus infection by an indirect enzyme-linked immunosorbent assay for specific immunoglobulin M (IgM) antibody without rheumatoid factor and specific IgG interference. J Clin Microbiol 1989;27:952-8.
19. Linde A, Kallin B, Dillner J, et al. Evaluation of enzyme-linked immunosorbent assays with two synthetic peptides of Epstein-Barr virus for diagnosis of infectious mononucleosis. J Infect Dis 1989;160:589-98.
20. Gray JJ. Avidity of EBV VCA-specific IgG antibodies: distinction between recent primary infection, past infection and reactivation. J Virol Methods 1995;52:95-104.
21. Edwards L, Ray CG, Meltzer P, Litwin CM, Sobonya RE, Chipowsky S Jr. Wasting disease associated with Epstein-Barr virus infection. Pediatr Infect Dis J 1988;7:719-24.
22. Buchwald D, Cheney PR, Peterson DL, et al. A chronic illness characterized by fatigue, neurologic and immunologic disorders, and active human herpesvirus type 6 infection. Ann Intern Med 1992;116:103-13.
23. Katz BZ, Raab-Traub N, Miller G. Latent and replicating forms of Epstein-Barr virus DNA in lymphomas and lymphoproliferative diseases. J Infect Dis 1989;160:589-98.
24. Muñoz FJ, Sharon N. Detection of human cytomegalovirus and Epstein-Barr virus in peripheral blood mononuclear cells with DNA probes. Laboratory Medicine 1990;21:742-5.
25. Okano M, Bashir RM, Davis JR, Purtilo DT. Detection of primary Epstein-Barr virus infection in a patient with X-linked lymphoproliferative disease receiving immunoglobulin prophylaxis. Am J Hematol 1991;36:294-6.
26. Peiper SC, Myers JL, Broussard EE, Sixbey JW. Detection of Epstein-Barr virus genomes in archival tissues by polymerase chain reaction. Arch Pathol Lab Med 1990;114:711-4.
27. Ambinder RF, Lambe BC, Mann RB, et al. Oligonucleotides for polymerase chain reaction amplification and hybridization detection of Epstein-Barr virus DNA in clinical specimens. Mol Cell Probes 1990;4:397-407.
28. Walter MA, Menarguez-Palanca J, Peiper SC. Epstein-Barr virus detection in neck metastases by polymerase chain reaction. Laryngoscope 1992;102:481-5.

29. Dictor M, Suven M, Tennvall J, Rambeck E. Determination of non-endemic nasopharyngeal carcinoma by *in situ* hybridization for Epstein-Barr virus EBER 1 RNA: sensitivity and specificity in cervical node metastasis. Laryngoscope 1995;105:407-12.
30. Saito I, Nishimura S, Kudo I, Fox RI, Moro I. Detection of Epstein-Barr virus and human herpes virus type 6 in saliva from patients with lymphoproliferative diseases by the polymerase chain reaction. Arch Oral Biol 1991;36:779-84.
31. Oda Y, Katsuda S, Okada Y, et al. Detection of human CMV, EBV and HSV in diffuse interstitial pneumonia by PCR and immunohistochemistry. Am J Clin Pathol 1994;102:495-502.

Human Immunodeficiency Viruses

Herminio R. Reyes, Ph.D.

Two distinct human immunodeficiency viruses, types 1 and 2 (HIV-1, -2), are the etiologic agents of AIDS.[1-3] AIDS due to HIV-1 infection is most prevalent in the Americas, Western Europe and Africa; whereas, most AIDS cases due to HIV-2 are reported in West Africa.[1-3] Phylogenetically, HIV-1 is divided into 9 subtypes (Group M [subtypes A-H] and Group O) and HIV-2 into 2 subtypes (A and B).[4] In Thailand, India and sub-Saharan Africa, ~90% of HIV-1 infections are acquired through heterosexual transmission in contrast with 10% in the U.S. and Western Europe.[2] Subtypes A, C and D predominate in Africa, subtypes E and B are commonly found in Thailand and C is the main subtype in India; whereas, subtype B predominates in the U.S. and Western Europe.[1,2] HIV-1 subtype E readily infects Langerhans' cells, which are particularly abundant in the cervical mucosa, and is implicated in facilitated transmission through heterosexual sex.[2] As of the end of 1995, the World Health Organization estimates that 18 million adults and 1.5 million children are infected with HIV resulting in ~4.5 million AIDS cases worldwide.[5]

In 50–93% of cases, primary HIV infection is symptomatic with a variety of symptoms ranging from influenza-like or mononucleosis-like illness to more severe neurological symptoms which can persist from a few days to as long as two months; longer acute clinical illness is associated with rapid progression to AIDS.[6,7] Rarely, progression to AIDS occurs rapidly but most individuals remain clinically asymptomatic for 1 to >10 years prior to clinical progression.[6] Other factors associated with rapid progression include oligoclonal expansion of CD8[+] T cells during acute infection[7] and high baseline viral load.[8]

Virus culture is the reference method for identifying HIV infection.[1] Positive culture rates of up to 98% are reported in confirmed seropositive individuals.[9] The culture method is, however, expensive, labor-intensive, can take weeks for complete results and potentially exposes laboratory workers to high concentrations of HIV.[1] Authoritative reviews on diagnostic tests, reference reagents, control values and guidelines for T lymphocyte subset enumeration in HIV-1 infection are available.[1,10-15]

Antibodies to HIV-1 are most commonly and reliably detected by EIA and confirmed by IB.[1] Antibody testing by EIA remains the standard method for screening potential blood donors; simultaneous testing for p24 antigenemia is superfluous.[16] Low risk potential donors with persistent, indeterminate immunoblots are rarely, if ever, infected with HIV.[17] Use of improved, third generation serological assays demonstrates that seroconversion typically occurs 3-12 weeks post-infection, although significant delays can occur in some individuals; p24 antigen positivity and/or PCR detection of proviral DNA further narrows the window period following primary infection.[18]

In diagnosing HIV-1 infection, the specificity of EIA is >99% when properly performed and the sensitivity is >98%.[1,19] In low-risk populations, the false-positive rate of combined EIA and IB testing is estimated to be <1 in 100,000 but the relatively high frequency (up to 20%) of indeterminate immunoblots in low-risk, EIA-positive individuals mandates improvement of confirmatory testing including IFA, radioimmunoprecipitation assay (RIPA), virus culture, PCR and EIA using recombinant viral envelope antigens.[1,20,21] Highly sensitive and specific agglutination and EIA methods for detection of type-specific antibodies to HIV-2 are available.[3,21] Inexpensive, sensitive and specific rapid format tests for HIV-specific antibodies[22,23] will be of great diagnostic value in developing nations where resources are limited and sophisticated laboratory technology is not widely available.

Causes of false-positive HIV EIAs[24]	Causes of false-negative HIV EIAs[24]
Hematologic malignant disorders	Window period prior to seroconversion
DNA viral infections	Immunosuppressive therapy
Autoimmune disorders	Replacement transfusion
Multiple myeloma	Malignant disorders
Primary biliary cirrhosis	B-cell dysfunction
Alcoholic hepatitis	Bone marrow transplantation
Influenza vaccination	Kits that primarily detect antibodies to p24
Hepatitis B vaccination	Laboratory glove starch powder
Passively transferred antibodies	
Antibodies to class II lymphocytes	
Renal transplantation	
Chronic renal failure	
Stevens-Johnson syndrome	
Positive RPR test	

EIA for HIV-1 antigen detects primarily uncomplexed p24 antigen,[25] is applicable to serum, plasma, CSF or cell culture,[26,27] indicates active infection,[26] can allow diagnosis before seroconversion,[28] can predict prognosis[29,30] and is useful for monitoring response to therapy.[31-33] Disadvantages of antigen detection assays include: poor sensitivity (only 69% in patients with AIDS[34] and as low as 20% in infants <1 month old[35]); detection is not possible in patients with a high titers of p24 antibody (which complexes with the antigen);[36] and failure to detect HIV-2 antigen.[37] The diagnostic and prognostic utility of measuring immune complex dissociated p24 antigen in plasma specimens remains controversial.[38-42] Antibodies to p24 antigen are a better predictive marker of progression than p24 antigen even after immune complex dissociation.[43]

PCR can detect proviral DNA in seronegative, high-risk or in seropositive, culture- and/or antigen-negative individuals, can differentiate latent HIV infection from active viral transcription and can quantitate the copy number of HIV DNA when used with external standards.[1,44-53] PCR can successfully differentiate between HIV-1 and HIV-2 infections.[54] Proviral DNA can be detected in peripheral blood mononuclear cells before seroconversion.[55,56] Limitations to the diagnostic use of PCR are rare false-negatives, some of which can be avoided by the use of multiple primer pairs and primers from conserved regions of the genome[57] and false-positives due to cross-contamination of the PCR reaction mixture.[58] Rapid PCR tests for detection of HIV DNA sequences applicable to the screening of blood donations from asymptomatic HIV-seronegative donors[59] (and perhaps in pooled clinical specimens) are promising for reliable mass screening of blood donations. Quantitation of

HIV RNA in plasma is useful for determining free viral load, assessing the efficacy of antiviral therapy and predicting progression and clinical outcome.[8,60-66] Because baseline HIV viral load is predictive of survival at 10 years in patients with nearly identical CD4[+] counts (70% survival with low viral load versus >70% mortality with high viral load),[61] assessment of baseline viremia prior to initiation of therapy is useful in patient management. RT-PCR has higher analytical sensitivity (100 copies/mL plasma) than branched-chain DNA detection (5,000-10,000 copies/mL plasma).[67-69]

Although transplacental transmission of HIV can occur as early at 8 weeks of gestation or possibly earlier, perinatal transmission of HIV-1 is said to result in >80% of AIDS cases in infants <1 year old.[1] Diagnosis of HIV-1 infection in infants born to seropositive mothers is difficult, because maternal IgG antibody to HIV-1 crosses the placenta and can persist for up to 15 months making the distinction between maternal and neonatal IgG difficult.[1] High maternal HIV RNA concentrations are predictive of vertical transmission and disease development in children infected *in utero* or during delivery.[1,58,67,70-72]

HIV-1 can be detected by PCR in the CSF of HIV-infected patients independently of disease stage; spread of HIV-1 to the brain represents an early event during infection which occurs in most asymptomatic individuals.[73] Intrathecal synthesis of HIV-specific IgG is reported in HIV-infected individuals who have ARC, AIDS or are asymptomatic.[74-77] Testing of CSF for HIV-specific IgG is useful diagnostically and prognostically because patients with neurologic symptoms including early AIDS dementia complex more frequently have these antibodies than asymptomatic patients.[75,78] Patients who present with aseptic meningitis and are at high risk for HIV infection should have both CSF and serum tested for HIV-1 antibodies because antibodies can appear in CSF before serum.[79] Measurement of HIV-1 antigens in CSF might have diagnostic and prognostic utility; preliminary studies indicate that antigen is present in CSF in most HIV-seropositive patients with focal or diffuse CNS pathologies.[80] PCR can detect proviral sequences (*gag* and *env*) in nucleated cells from antigen-negative CSF of HIV-1 seropositive individuals; up to 95% of such individuals can have neurologic abnormalities.[81] The percentage of AIDS patients with HIV encephalopathy is highest in individuals younger than 15 years and those older than 60 years[82] (the age groups in whom the immune system is normally suboptimal); this distribution of HIV encephalopathy is consistent with an infectious etiology. The treatment- and age-adjusted relative risk for accelerated progression in patients with neurologic manifestations of primary HIV infection is >2-fold higher than that of patients without neurologic manifestations.[83] A review of the clinical features, pathogenic mechanisms and treatment of neurologic manifestations of HIV infection is available.[84]

Prognostic factors for progression to AIDS requiring further study include elevated serum prolactin concentrations,[85] decreased dehydroepiandrosterone concentrations,[86] the presence of antibodies to HIV-1 virion infectivity factor (*vif*) protein,[87] decreased serum HIV-1 reverse transcriptase-specific antibodies,[88] and elevated serum IgE concentrations.[89] The role of cytokines and cytokine receptors and their potential prognostic value in HIV infection also require further investigation.[90,91] Early HIV-1 infection is characterized by type 2 cytokine production and lymphocyte activation (e.g., reduced mitogen-stimulated IL-2 and IFN-γ production, increased mitogen-stimulated IL-4 and IL-10 production, a relative decrease in CD4[+] and CD4[+]/CD7[-] and an increase in CD4[+]CD7[-]CD57[+] lymphocytes, and a relative increase in CD8[+], CD8[+]CD38[+] and CD8[+]CD57[+] lymphocytes), and closely resembles advanced HIV infection.[90] Patients with cytotropic syncytium-inducing HIV-1 isolates have a higher relative risk of disease progression independently of low CD4[+] counts or p24 antigenemia.[92,93]

Mutations in the HIV *pol* gene are associated with resistance to the antiretroviral agents ZDV, ddI, 3TC and d4T and correlate with clinical progression as defined by commonly accepted clinical endpoints such as development of a new opportunistic infection or death.[94-101] Resistance to protease inhibitors also occurs, albeit more slowly when used in combination with nucleoside analogs.[102-105] Therefore, phenotypic drug resistance studies and detection of specific mutations can be a useful adjunct to therapeutic decision-making. DNA sequencing is the most direct and sensitive method for evaluating point mutations.

Recent reviews of the biology, life cycle, genomic organization and regulation of replication of human immunodeficiency viruses,[106] the immunopathogenesis of HIV infection[107-109] and of the evaluation and treatment of the late sequelae of HIV infection[110,111] are available. Well-defined guidelines for minimizing the impact of opportunistic infections in HIV-infected patients[112-114] and recommendations for investigative studies of surrogate markers[115] are also available. Efficacy trials of HIV vaccines will require screening assays which distinguish uninfected vaccine recipients from HIV-infected individuals and which can detect different HIV subtypes.[2,116-119] Kinetic studies of viral clearance and loss of virus producing cells,[120] which reveal an average half life of productively infected cells of 1.6 days and an estimated average total HIV-1 production of 10.3×10^9 virions per day, should enable development of treatment strategies to block *de novo* HIV-1 replication. See Chapter 2: *Streptococcus pneumoniae.*

REFERENCES

1. Hu DJ, Dondero TJ, Rayfield MA, et al. The emerging genetic diversity of HIV. The importance of global surveillance for diagnostics, research and prevention. JAMA 1996;275:210-6.
2. Dillner L. HIV subtype may explain sexual transmission [News]. Br Med J 1996;312:530-1.
3. Imai M, Hayashi T, Kondo M, et al. Differentiation of human immunodeficiency virus type 1 (HIV-1) infections from HIV-2-cross-reacting antibody from mixed infections with HIV-1 and HIV-2 by serological absorption test. J Clin Microbiol 1995;33:1727-9.
4. Gürtler LG, Zekeng L, Simon F, et al. Reactivity of five anti-HIV-1 subtype O specimens with six different anti-HIV screening ELISAs and three immunoblots. J Virol Methods 1995;51:177-84.
5. Centers for Disease Control and Prevention. First 500,000 AIDS cases - United States, 1995. JAMA 1995;274:1827-8.
6. Roos MTL, Lange JMA, de Goede REY. Viral phenotype and immune response in primary human immunodeficiency virus type 1 infection. J Infect Dis 1992;165:427-32.
7. Pantaleo G. Virologic and immunologic events associated with primary HIV infection, pp. 655-7. In: Fauci AS, moderator. Immunopathogenic mechanisms of HIV infection. Ann Intern Med 1996;124:654-63.
8. Mellors J, et al. 3rd National Conference on Retroviruses and Opportunistic Infections. Washington, D.C., January, 1996 [News in: Science 1996;271:755-6].
9. Jackson JB, Kwok SY, Sninksy JJ, et al. Human immunodeficiency virus type 1 detected in all seropositive symptomatic and asymptomatic individuals. J Clin Microbiol 1990;28:16-9.
10. Bylund DJ, Ziegner UHM, Hooper DG. Review of testing for human immunodeficiency virus. Clin Lab Med 1992;12:305-33.
11. Glassman AB. Human immunodeficiency virus: testing and interpretation. Infectious Diseases Newsletter 1992;11:41-3.
12. Raboud JM, Haley L, Montaner JSG, Murphy C, Januszewska M, Schechter MT. Quantification of the variation due to laboratory and physiologic sources in CD4 lymphocyte counts of clinically stable HIV-infected individuals. J Acquir Immune Defic Syndr Human Retrovirol 1995;10:S67-73.
13. Centers for Disease Control. Guidelines for the performance of CD4+ T-cell determinations in persons with human immunodeficiency virus infection. MMWR Morbid Mortal Wkly Rep 1992;41:1-17.
14. Bootman JS, Kitchin PA. An international collaborative study to assess a set of reference reagent for HIV-1 PCR. J Virol Methods 1992;37:23-42.
15. Johnson D, Hirschkorn D, Busch MP, et al. Evaluation of four alternative methodologies for determination of absolute CD4+ lymphocyte counts. J Acquir Immune Defic Syndr Hum Retrovirol 1995;10:522-30.
16. Alter HJ, Epstein JS, Swneson SG, et al. Prevalence of human immunodeficiency virus type 1 p24 antigen in U.S. blood donors - an assessment ofthe efficacy of testing in donor screening. N Engl J Med 1990;323:1312-7.
17. Jackson JB, MacDonald KL, Cadwell J, et al. Absence of HIV infection in blood donors with indeterminate Western blot tests for antibody to HIV-1. N Engl J Med 1990;322:217-22.

18. Busch MP, Lee LLL, Satten GA, et al. Time course of detection of viral and serologic markers preceding human immunodeficiency virus type 1 seroconversion: implications for screening of blood and tissue donors. Transfusion 1995;35:91-7.

19. Matter L, Germann D. Detection of human immunodeficiency virus (HIV) type 1 antibodies by new automated microparticle enzyme immunoassay for HIV types 1 and 2. J Clin Microbiol 1995;33:2338-41.

20. Celum CL, Coombs RW, Jones M, et al. Risk factors for repeatedly reactive HIV-1 EIA and indeterminate western blots. Arch Intern Med 1994;154:1129-37.

21. Nuwayhid NF. Laboratory test for detection of human immunodeficiency virus type 1 infection. Clin Diagn Lab Immunol 1995;2:637-45.

22. Asihene PJ, Kline RL, Moss MW, Carella AV, Quinn TC. Evaluation of rapid test for detection of antibody to human immunodeficiency virus type 1 and type 2. J Clin Microbiol 1994;32:1341-2.

23. Jayaraman KS. India refining simple HIV test [News]. Nature Med 1995;1:984.

24. Cordes RJ, Ryan ME. Pitfalls in HIV testing. Application ans limitations of current tests. Postgrad Med 1995;98:177-89.

25. Goudsmit J, Lange JMA, Paul DA, Dawson GJ. Antigenemia and antibody titers to core and envelope antigens in AIDS, AIDS-related complex, and subclinical human immunodeficiency virus infection. J Infect Dis 1987;155:558-60.

26. Jackson JB. Human immunodeficiency virus type 1 antigen and culture assays. Arch Pathol Lab Med 1990;114:249-53.

27. Singer EJ, Syndulko K, Fahy-Chandon BN, et al. Cerebrospinal fluid p24 antigen levels and intrathecal immunoglobuling G synthesis are associated with cognitive disease severity in HIV-1. AIDS 1994;8:197-204.

28. Kingsley LA, Rinaldo C, Gupta R, et al. The temporal relationship between HIV p24 antigenemia and HIV seroconversion [Abstract]. Fourth International Conference on AIDS. Stockholm, Sweden: 1988.

29. Moss AR, Bacchetti P, Osmond D, et al. Seropositivity for HIV and the development of AIDS or AIDS related condition: three year follow up of the San Francisco General Hospital cohor. Br Med J 1988;296:745-50.

30. Farley JJ, Bauer G, Johnson JP, Cole GA. Phytohemagglutinin-inducible p24 in peripheral blood mononuclear cells as a predictor of human immunodeficiency virus type 1 vertical transmission and infant clinical status. Pediatr Inf Dis J 1994;13:1079-82.

31. Chaisson RE, Allain J-P, Luther M, Volderding PA. Monocytes in AIDS [Letter]. N Engl J Med 1986;315:1610-1.

32. Jackson CG, Paul DA, Falk LA, et al. Human immunodeficiency virus (HIV) antigenemia (p24) in the acquired immunodeficiency syndrome (AIDS) and the effect of treatment with zidovudine (AZT). Ann Intern Med 1988;108:175-80.

33. Studies of Ocular Complications of AIDS Research Group in collaboration with AIS Clinical Trials Group. Antiviral effects of foscarnet and ganciclovir therapy on human immunodeficiency virus p24 antigen in patients with AIDS and cytomegalovirus retinitis. J Infect Dis 1995;172:613-21.

34. Paul DA, Falk LA, Kessler HA, et al. Correlation of serum HIV antigen and antibody with clinical status in HIV-infected patients. J Med Virol 1987;22:357-63.

35. Andiman WA, Silva TJ, Shapiro ED, O'Connor T, Olson B. Predictive value of the human immunodeficiency virus 1 antigen test in children born to infected mothers. Pediatr Infect Dis J 1992;11:436-40.

36. McHugh TM, Stites DP, Busch MP, et al. Relation of circulating levels of human immunodeficiency virus (HIV) antigen, antibody to p24, and HIV-containing immune complexes in HIV-infected patients. J Infect Dis 1988;158:1088-91.

37. Paul D, Knigge M, Kennedy M, Mack D, Leibowitch J. Detection of HIV-2 Ag in serum and culture by HIV-1 Ag EIA [Abstract]. Fourth International Conference on AIDS. Stockholm, Sweden: 1988.

38. Lewis DE, Adu-Oppong A, Hollinger FB, et al. Sensitivity of immune complex-dissociated p24 antigen testing for early detection of human immunodeficiency virus in infants. ClinDiagn Lab Immunol 1995;2:87-90.

39. Bulterys M, Farzadegan H, Chao A, et al. Diagnostic utility of immune-complex-dissociated p24 antigen detection in perinatally acquired HIV-1 infection in Rwanda. J Acquir Immune Defic Syndr Hum Retrovirol 1995;10:186-91.

40. Duiculescu DC, Geffin RB, Scott GB, Scott WA. Clinical and immunological correlates of immune-complex-dissociated HIV-1 p24 antigen in HIV-1-infected children. J Acquir Immune Defic Syndr 1994;7:807-15.

41. Rodríguez-Iglesias MA, Alvarez JR, Vergara A, Garcia-Valdivia MS, Jesús I, Mira J. Improved detection of HIV p24 antigen in serum after acid pretreatment. Eur J Clin Microbiol Infect Dis 1992;11:849-50.

42. Miles SA, Balden E, Magpantay L, et al. Rapid serologic testing with immune-complex-dissociated HIV p24 antigen for early detection of HIV infection in neonates. NEJM 1993;328:297-302.

43. Morand-Joubert L, Bludau H, Lerable J, Petit JC, Lefrère JJ. Serum anti-p24 antibody concentration has a predictive value on the decrease of CD4 lymphocyte count higher than acid-dissociated p24 antigen. J Med Virol 1995;47:87-91.

44. Loussert-Ajaka I, Simon F, Farfara I, et al. Comparative study of simgle and nested PCR for the detection of proviral HIV2 DNA. Res Virol 1994;145:337-42.

45. Hsia K, Tsai V, Zvaifler NJ, Spector SA. Low prevalence of HIV-1 proviral DNA in peripheral blood monocytes and dendritic cells from HIV-1-infected individuals. AIDS 1995;9:398-9.

46. Brossard Y, Aubin J-T, Mandelbrot L, et al. Frequency of early *in utero* HIV-1 infection: a blind DNA polymerase chain reaciton study on 100 fetal thymuses. AIDS 1995;9:359-66.

47. Janssens W, Fransen K, Loussert-Ajaka I, et al. Diagnosis of HIV-1 group O infection by polymerase chain reaction. Lancet 1995;346:451-2.

48. Kovacs A, Xu J, Rasheed S, et al. Comparison of a rapid nonisotopic polymerase chain reaction assay with four commonly used methods for the early diagnosis of human immunodeficiency virus type 1 infection in neonates and children. Pediatr Infect Dis J 1995;14:948-54.

49. Bagasra O, Farzadegan H, Seshamma T, Oakes JW, Saah A, Pomerant RJ. Detection of HIV-1 proviral DNA in sperm from HIV-1-infected men. AIDS 1994;8:1669-74.

50. Sethoe SY, Ling AE, Sng EH, Montiero EH, Chan RKW. PCR as a confirmatory test for human immunodeficiency virus type 1 infection in individuals with indeterminate western blot (immunoblot) profiles. J Clin Microbiol 1995;33:3034-6.

51. Peckham C, Gibb D. Mother-to-child transmission of the human immunodeficiency virus. NEJM 1995;333:298-302.

52. Newell M-L, Dunn D, De Maria A, et al. Detection of virus in vertically exposed HIV-antibody-negative children. Lancet 1996;347:213-5.

53. Zella D, Cavicchini A, Cattaneo E, Cimarelli A, Bertazzoni U. Utilization of a DNA enzyme immunoassay for the detection of proviral DNA of human immunodeficiency virus type 1 by polymerase chain reaction. Clin Diagn Virol 1995;3:155-64.

54. Rayfield M, De Cock D, Heward W, et al. Mixed human immunodeficiency virus (HIV) infection in an individual: demonstration of both HIV type 1 and type 2 proviral sequences by using polymerase chain reaction. J Infect Dis 1988;158:1170-6.

55. Gorriño MT, Campelo C, Suarez MD, Santamaría A, Malave C, Cisterna R. Detection of human immunodeficiency virus type 1 by PCR before seroconversion in high-risk individuals who remain seronegative for prolonged periods. Eur J Clin Microbiol Infect Dis 1994;13:271-6.

56. Bruisten SM, Mientjes GHC, van Delft P, et al. HIV-1 infection detected by polymerase chain reaction frequently precedes antibody seroconversion in drug users. AIS 1994;8:1736-7.

57. Ou C-Y, Kwok S, Mitchell SW, et al. DNA amplification for direct detection of HIV-1 in DNA of peripheral blood mononuclear cells. Science 1988;239:295-7.

58. Dickover RE, Garratty EM, Herman SA, et al. Identification of levels of maternal HIV-1 RNA associated with risk of perinatal transmission. Effect of maternalzidovudine treatment on viral load. JAMA 1996;275:599-605.

59. Sevall JS, Prince H, Garratty G, O'Brien WA, Zack JA. Rapid enzymatic analysis for HIV-1 DNA in clinical specimens. Clin Chem 1993;39:433-9.

60. Richman DD. Drug resistance in relation to pathogenesis. AIDS 1995;9:S49-53.

61. Kappes JC, Saag MS, Shaw GM, et al. Assessment of antiretroviral therapy by plasma viral load testing: standard and ICD HIV-1 p24 antigen and viral RNA (QC-PCR) assays compared. J Acquir Immune Def Syndr 1995;10:139-49.

62. Ruffault A, Michelet C, Jacquelinet C, et al. The prognostic value of plasma viremia in HIV-infected patients under AZT treatment: a two-year follow-up study. J Acquir Immune Defic Syndr 1995;9:243-8.

63. Rinaldo C, Huang X-L, Fan Z, et al. High levels of anti-human immunodeficiency virus type 1 (HIV-1) memory cytotoxic T-lymphocyte activity and low viral load are associated with lack of disease in HIV-1-infected long-term nonprogressors. J Virol 1995;69:5838-42.

64. Merigan TC, Hirsch RL, Fisher AC, Meyerson LA, Glodstein G, Winters MA. The prognostic significance of serum viral load, codon 215 reverse transcriptase mutation and CD4+ T cells on progression of HIV disease in a double-blind study of thymopentin. AIDS 1996;10:159-65.

65. Katzenstein TL, Pedersen C, Nielsen C, Lundgren JD, Jakobsen PH, Gerstoft J. Longitudinal serum HIV RNA quantification: correlation to viral phenotype at seroconversion and clinical outcome. AIDS 1996;10:167-73.

66. Bush CE, Donovan RM, Markowitz N, Baxa D, Kvale P, Saravolatz LD. Gender is nor a factor in serum human immunodeficiency virus type 1 RNA levels in patients with viremia. J Clin Microbiol 1996;34:970-2.

67. Volberding PA. HIV quantification: clinical applications. Lancet 1996;347:71-3.

68. Piatak M Jr, Saag MS, Yang LC, et al. Determination of plasma viral load in HIV-1 infection by quantitative competitive polymerase chain reaction. AIDS 1993;7:S65-71.

69. Angeles Muñoz-Fernández M, Navarro J, García Montes M, Cosín J, Zabay JM, Fernández-Cruz E. Quantification of low levels of human immunodeficiency virus (HIV) type 1 RNA in p24 antigen-negative, asymptomatic, HIV-positive patients by PCR. J Clin Microbiol 1996;34:404-8.

70. Mayaux M-J, Burgard M, Teglas J-P, et al. Neonatal characteristics in rapidly progressive perinatally acquired HIV-1 disease. JAMA 1996;275:606-10.

71. Fang G, Burger H, Grimson R, et al. Maternal plasma human immunodeficiency virus type 1 RNA level: A determinant and projected threshold for mother-to-child transmission. PNAS USA 1995;92:12,100-04.

72. DeRossi A, Masiero S, Giaquinto C, et al. Dynamics of viral replication in infants with vertically acquired human immunodeficiency virus type 1 infection. J Clin Invest 1996;97:323-30.

73. Chiodi F, Keys B, Albert J, et al. Human immunodeficiency virus type 1 is present in the cerebrospinal fluid of a majority of infected individuals. J Clin Microbiol 1992;30:1768-71.

74. Goudsmit J, Wolters EC, Bakker M, et al. Intrathecal synthesis of antibodies to HTLV-III in patients without AIDS or AIDS related complex. Br Med J 1986;292:1231-4.

75. Resnick L, DiMarzo-Veronese F, Schüpbach J, et al. Intra-blood-brain-barrier synthesis of HTLV-III specific IgG in patients with neurologic symptoms associated with AIDS or AIDS-related complex. N Engl J Med 1985;313:1498-504.

76. Van Wielink G, McArthur JC, Moench T, et al. Intrathecal synthesis of anti-HIV IgG: correlation with increasing duration of HIV-1 infection. Neurology 1990;40:816-9.

77. Hall CD, Snyder CR, Robertson KR, et al. Cerebrospinal fluid analysis in human immunodeficiency virus infection. Ann Clin Lab Sci 1992;22:139-43.

78. Elovaara I, Seppälä I, Poutiainen E, Suni J, Valle S-L. Intrathecal humoral immunologic response in neurologically symptomatic and asymptomatic patients with human immunodeficiency virus infection. Neurology 1988;38:1451-5.

79. Rolfs A, Schumacher HC. Early findings in the cerebrospinal fluid of patients with HIV-1 infection of the central nervous system. N Engl J Med 1990;323:418-9.

80. Scalzini A, Scura G, Stellini R, Cristini G. HIV1-Ag in cerebrospinal fluid during AIDS. Acta Neurol 1990;12:53-7.

81. Shaunak S, Albright RE, Klotman ME, Henry SC, Bartlett JA, Hamilton JD. Amplification of HIV-1 provirus from cerebrospinal fluid and its correlation with neurologic disease. J Infect Dis 1990;161:1068-72.

82. Janssen RS, Nwanyanwu OC, Selik RM, Stehr-Green JK. Epidemiology of human immunodeficiency virus encephalopathy in the United States. Neurology 1992;42:1472-6.

83. Boufassa F, Bachmeyer C, Carré N, et al. Influence of neurologic manifestations of primary human immunodeficiency virus infection on disease progression. J Infect Dis 1995;171:1190-5.

84. Simpson DM, Tagliati M. Neurologic manifestations of HIV infection. Ann Intern Med 1994;121:769-85.

85. Graef AS, Gonzalez SS, Baca VR, et al.. High serum prolactin levels in asymptomatic HIV-infected patients and in patients with acquired immunodeficiency syndrome. Clin Immunol Immunopathol 1994;72:390-3.

86. Mulder JW, Jos Frissen PH, Krijnen P, et al. Dehydroepiandrosterone as predictor for progression to AIDS in asymptomatic human immunodeficiency virus-infected men. J Infect Dis 1992;165:413-8.

87. Schwander S, Braun RW, Kühn JE, et al. Prevalence of antibodies to recombinant virion infectivity factor in the sera of prospectively studied patients with HIV-1 infection. J Med Virol 1992;36:142-6.

88. Neumüller M, Karlsson A, Lennerstrand J, et al. HIV-1 reverse transcriptase inhibiting antibody titer in serum: Relation to disease progression and to core-antibody levels. J Med Virol 1992;36:283-91.

89. Ellaurie M, Rubinstein A, Rosenstreich DL. IgE levels in pediatric HIV-1 infection. Ann Allergy Asthma Immunol 1995;75:332-6.

90. Meroni L, Trabattoni D, Balotta C, et al. Evidence for type 2 cytokine production and lymphocyte activation in the early phases of HIV-1 infection. AIDS 1996;10:23-30.

91. Marfaing-Koka A, Aubin J-T, Grangeot-Keros L, et al. In vivo role of IL-6 on the viral load and on immunological abnormalities of HIV-infected patients. J Acquir Immune Defic Syndr Hum Retrovirol 1996;11:59-68.

92. Todd BJ, Kedar P, Pope JH. Syncytium induction in primary CD4+ T-cell lines from normal donors by human immunodeficiency virus type 1 isolates with non-syncytium-inducing genotype and phenotype in MT-2 cells. J Virol 1995;69:7099-105.

93. Fouchier RAM, Brouwer M, Broersen SM, Schuitemaker H. Simple determination of human immunodeficiency virus type 1 syncytium-inducing V3 genotype by PCR. J Clin Microbiol 1995;33:906-11.

94. Frenkel LM, Wagner LE, Atwood SM, Cummins TJ, Dewhurst S. Specific, sensitive, and rapid assay for human immunodeficiency virus type 1 *pol* mutations associated with resistance to zidovudine and didanosine. J Clin Microbiol 1995;33:342-7.

95. Di Stefano M, Sabri F, Leitner T, et al. Reverse transcriptase sequence of paired isolates of cerebrospinal fluid and blood from patients infected with human immunodeficiency virus type 1 during zidovudine treatment. J Clin Microbiol 1995;33:352-5.

96. Holodniy M, Mole L, Margolis D, et al. Determination of human immunodeficiency virus RNA in plasma and cellular viral DNA genotypic zidovudine resistance and viral load during zidovudine-didanosine combination therapy. J Virol 1995;69:3510-6.

97. Goulden MG, Cammack N, Hopewell PL, Penn CR, Cameron JM. Selection *in vitro* of an HIV-1 variant resistant to both lamivudine (3TC) and zidovudine. AIDS 1996;10:101-2.

98. Wainberg MA, Salomon H, Gu Z, et al. Development of HIV-1 resistance to (-)2'-deoxy-3'-thiacitidine in patients with AIDS or advance AIDS-related complex. AIDS 1995;9:351-7.

99. Kavlick MF, Shirasaka T, Kojima E, et al. Genotypic and phenotypic characterization of HIV-1 isolated from patients receiving (-)-2'-3'-dideoxy-3'-thiacitidine. Antiviral Res 1995;28:133-46.

100. D'Aquila RT. HIV-1 chemotherapy and drug resistance. Clin Diagn Virol 1995;3:299-316.

101. Gu Z, Gao Q, Salomon H, Wainberg MA. A novel mutation at codon 50 in the HIV-1 pol gene that encodes resistance to 2', 3'-didehydro-3'-deoxythymidine (d4T). Natlional Conference on Human Retroviruses and Related Infection (1st), December 12-16, 1993.

102. Richman DD. Protease uninhibited. Nature 1995;374:494.

103. Condra JH, Schleif WA, Blahy OM, et al. *In vivo* emergence of HIV-1 variants resistant to multiple protease inhibitors. Nature 1995;374:569-71.

104. Winslow DL, Otto MJ. HIV protease inhibitors. AIDS 1995;9:S183-92.

105. Roberts NA. Drug-resistance patterns of saquinavir and other HIV proteinase inhibitors. AIDS 1995;9:S27-32.

106. Bryant ML, Ratner L. Biology and molecular biology of human immunodeficiency virus. Pediatr Infect Dis J 1992;11:390-400.

107. Fauci AS. Immunopathogenic mechanisms of HIV infection. Ann Intern Med 1996;124:654-63.

108. Schellekens PTA, Koot M, Roos MTL, Tersmette M, Miedema F. Immunologic and virologic markers determining progression to AIDS. J Acquir Immune Defic Syndr Hum Retrovirol 1995;10:S62-6.

109. Lewin SR, Crowe SM. AIDS pathogenesis. AIDS 1994;8:S3-11.

110. Northfelt DW. Evaluation and treatment of the later manifestations of HIV infection. Prim Care 1992;19:57-85.

111. Fauci A. Immunopathogenic mechanisms of human immunodeficiency virus disease: implications for therapy. Am J Med 1995;99:59S-60S.

112. Kaplan JE, Masur H, Jaffe HW, Holmes KK. Reducing the impact of opportunistic infections in patients with HIV infection. New guidelines. JAMA 1995;274:347-8.

113. Kaplan JE, Masur H, Holmes KK, et al. USPHS/IDSA guidelines for the prevention of opportunistic infections in persons infected with human immunodeficiency virus: Introduction. Clin Infect Dis 1995;21:S1-11.

114. Kaplan JE, Masur H, Holmes KK, et al. USPHS/IDSA guidelines for the prevention of opportunistic infections in persons infected with human immunodeficiency virus: An overview. Clin Infect Dis 1995;21:S12-31.

115. Scientific Advisory Committee on Surrogate Markers of HIV. Consensus statement. J Acquir Immune Defic Syndr Hum Retrovirol 1995;10:S114-6.

116. Schwartz DH, Mazumdar A, Winston S, Harkonen S. Utility of various commercially available human immunodeficiency virus (HIV) antibody diagnostic kits for use in conjunction with efficacy trials of HIV-1 vaccines. Clin Diagn Lab Immunol 1995;2:268-71.

117. Hanson CV. Measuring vaccine-induced HIV neutralization: report of a workshop. AIDS Res Hum Retroviruses 1994;10:645-8.

118. Belshe RB, Graham BS, Keefer MC, et al. Neutralizing antibodies to HIV-1 in seronegative volunteers immunized with recombinant gp120 from the MN strain of HIV-1. JAMA 1994;272:475-80.

119. Mascola JR, McNeil JG, Burke DS. AIDS vaccines. Are we ready for human efficacy trials? JAMA 1994;272:488-9.

120. Perelson AS, Neumann AU, Markowitz M, Leonard JM, Ho DD. HIV-1 dynamics in vivo: virion clearance rate, infected cell life-span, and viral generation time. Science 1996;271:1582-6.

Parainfluenza Virus

Pamela Bean, Ph.D.

Three related single stranded RNA paramixoviruses, collectively called parainfluenza viruses (PIVs) type 1, 2 and 3, cause appreciable respiratory morbidity each year among infants and young children.[1] The clinical manifestations of parainfluenza virus infection, croup, upper respiratory infections and pharyngitis, were recently identified in pediatric organ transplant recipients.[2]   By EIA, increases in IgG antibodies to PIV are detected in at least 93%, 81% and 80% of PIV type 1, 2 and 3 infections, respectively; IgM antibodies are found in 40-90%.[3]   Cross-reactions of IgG antibodies to PIV 1 and 3 are common, but not of antibodies to PIV 2 with PIV 1 and 3; cross-reactions are less frequent (26–36%) with IgM responses.[3,4]   EIA is more sensitive than CF, but of lower specificity because cross-reactions of PIV with mumps virus occur.[5]   Type-specific PIV antigens are detectable in 94–100% of culture-positive nasopharyngeal aspirates.[6]   PIV 3 was identified by HI and IFA in CSF from patients with symptoms suggestive of meningitis.[7]   DNA probe and PCR techniques can discriminate between between PIV and measles virus in subacute sclerosing panencephalitis (SSPE).[8]

REFERENCES

1. Knott AM, Long CE, Hall CB. Parainfluenza viral infections in pediatric outpatients: seasonal patterns and clinical characteristics. Pediatr Infect Dis J 1994;13:269-73.
2. Apalsch AM, Green M, Ledesma-Medina J, Nour B, Wald ER. Parainfluenza and influenza virus infections in pediatric organ transplant recipients. Clin Infect Dis 1995;20:394-9.
3. Vuorinen T, Meurman O.   Enzyme immunoassays for detection of IgG and IgM antibodies to parainfluenza types 1, 2 and 3. J Virol Methods 1989;23:63-70.
4. Ray R, Matsuoka Y, Burnett TL, Glaze BJ, Compnas RW. Human parainfluenza virus induces a type-specific protective immune response. J Infect Dis 1990;162:746-9.
5. Fraňková V, Holubová J, Grubhoffer L, Kašová V. Contribution to laboratory diagnosis of mumps and parainfluenza. Acta Virol (Praha) 1988;32:503-14.
6. Hierholzer JC, Bingham PG, Coombs RA, Johansson KH, Anderson LJ, Halonen PE.   Comparison of monoclonal antibody time-resolved fluoroimmunoassay with monoclonal antibody capture-biotinylated detector enzyme immunoassay for respiratory syncytial virus and parainfluenza virus antigen detection. J Clin Microbiol 1989;27:1234-9.
7. Vreede RW, Schellekens H, Zuijderwijk M. Isolation of parainfluenza virus type 3 from cerebrospinal fluid [Letter]. J Infect Dis 1992;165:1166.
8. Baram TZ, Gonzales-Gomez I, Xie ZD, et al.   Subacute sclerosing panencephalitis in an infant: diagnostic role of viral genome analysis. Ann Neurol 1995;36:103-8.

Parvovirus B19

J. Sanders Sevall, Ph.D.

Parvovirus B19, a single-stranded DNA virus,[1] is the only parvovirus with an identified role in the pathogenesis of human disease.[2]   During viremia (~7 to 10 days post-exposure) the B19 virus destroys erythroid precursor cells, compromising red blood cell production and causing transient aplastic crisis in patients with chronic hemolytic anemias.[3] IgM antibodies to parvovirus B19 begin to circulate at high titer during the second week after exposure. Chronic parvovirus B19 infection in patients with immunodeficiency can lead to bone marrow erythropoietic failure.[4] Prompt recognition of persistent B19 is important, not only because it can be treated with intravenous immunoglobulin but also to prevent nosocomial transmission to other immunocompromised patients.[5,6] The prevalence of antibodies to parvovirus B19 is 60% or more in adults without evidence of hematological disease and indicates that infection is acquired during childhood.[7] In erythema infectiosum, a rubella-like illness with malar rash (also known as fifth disease), adult flu-like symptoms and arthropathies begin coincident with IgG antibody production (~18 days post exposure) and are probably immune-complex mediated.[3]   In adults, especially women, infection is often complicated by acute arthritis and other rheumatologic manifestations.[8-10]   Acute parvovirus infection can occur during pregnancy but an adverse fetal outcome is a rare complication.[11,12] However, parvovirus B19 was detected in 66% of the pediatric patients who presented with non-A, non-B fulminant liver failure and associated aplastic anemia.[13]

Culture techniques[14] and the cloning of parvovirus B19 structural proteins and their expression in recombinant DNA systems have greatly increased the availability of antibody detection assays.[15-17]   A variety of antibody assays including EIA, antibody capture RIA and immunoblot can be used to detect IgM antibodies to parvovirus B19 (current/recent infection) or rise in titer of IgG antibodies (recent infection) or presence of IgG antibodies (immune status).[18,19] Markers of acute parvovirus B19 infection in serum of persons with erythema infectiosum tested by capture EIA reveal specific IgM antibodies are the most sensitive indicator and persist up to 6 months; IgA antibodies are too persistent to be a useful marker of recent B19 infection. B19 DNA can often be detected up to 2 months after onset of illness and can be useful for diagnosis of acute B19 infection.[20] Low level or equivocal results (not serological cross-reactivity) are reported in early tests for rubella antibodies in serum with high titers of parvovirus IgM and in tests for parvovirus in serum with high titers of rubella IgM.[21] Increased antibody specificity in more recent investigations have increased the utility of both IgM and IgG for accurate serodiagnosis of recent parvovirus infections.[22,23] Both antibody and DNA testing are recommended for detecting parvovirus B19 infection in the immunocompromised, in chronic anemics and in fetal tissue/amniotic fluid.[5,24] PCR, the most sensitive method for detecting parvovirus B19 DNA in urine, amniotic fluid, pleural fluid, synovial fluid and serum,[25,26] can reveal B19 DNA in patients who have not yet developed specific IgM and IgG antibodies and in some sera even when specific IgM and/or IgG are present. PCR detection of parvovirus B19 in amniotic fluid is promising for identification of fetuses at high risk.[27] Using a hemagglutination test for screening blood donors, B19 antigen can be detected in high titer ($\geq 10^8$ genomes/μL) donated blood.[28] A comprehensive review on parvovirus B19 for the hematologist is available.[29]

REFERENCES

1. Berns KI. Parvovirus replication. Microbiol Rev 1990;54:316-29.
2. Cohen B. Parvovirus B19: an epanding spectrum of disease. Br Med J 1995;311:1549-52.
3. Anderson LJ. Human parvoviruses. J Infect Dis 1990;161:603-8.
4. Frickhofen N, Abkowitz JL, Safford M, et al. Persistent B19 parvovirus infection in patients infected with human immunodeficiency virus type 1 (HIV-1): a treatable cause of anemia in AIDS. Ann Intern Med 1990;113:926-33.
5. Sevall JS, Rittenhouse JW, Peter JB. Laboratory diagnosis of parvovirus B19 infection. J Clin Anal 1992;6:171-5.
6. Evans JPM, Rossiter MA, Kumarian TO, Marsh GW, Mortimer PP. Human parvovirus aaplasia: case due to cross infection in a ward. B Med J 1984;288:681.
7. Cohen BJ, Buckley MM. The prevalence of antibody to human parvovirus B19 in England and Wales. J Med Microbiol 1988;25:151-3.
8. Gran JT, Johnsen V, Nordbø SA. The variable clinical picture of arthritis induced by human parvovirus. Scand J Rheumatol 1995;24:174-9.
9. Naides SJ, Scharosch LL, Foto F, Howard EJ. Rheumatologic manifestations of human parvovirus B19 infection in adults. Initial two-year clinical experience. Arthritis Rheum 1990;33:1297-309.
10. Garcia-Tapian AM, Fernandez-Gutierrez C, Giron JA, et al. Spectrum of parovirus B19 infection: analysis of an outbreak of 43 cases in Cadiz, Spain. Clin Infect Dis 1995:21:1424-39.
11. Hall SM, Cohn BJ, Mortimer PP, et al. Prospective study of human parvovirus (B19) infection in pregnancy. Br Med J 1990;300:1166-70.
12. Gratacos E, Torres PJ, Vidal J, et al. The incidence of human parvovirus B19 infection during pregnancy and its impact on perinatal outcome. J Infect Dis 1995;171:1360-3.
13. Langnas AN, Markin RS, Cattral MS, et al. Parvovirus B19 as a possible causative agent of fulminant liver failure and associated aplastic anemia. Hepatology 1995;22:1661-5.
14. Shimomura S, Komatsu N, Frickhofen N, Anderson S, Kajigaya S, Young NS. First continuous propagation of B19 parvovirus in a cell line. Blood 1992;79:18-24.
15. Sisk WP, Berman ML. Expression of human parvovirus B19 structural protein in E. coli and detection of antiviral antibodies in human serum. Biotechnology 1987;5:1077-80.
16. Kajigaya S, Fujii H, Field A, et al. Self-assembled B19 parvovirus capsids, produced in a baculovirus system, are antigenically and immunogenically similar to native virions. Proc Natl Acad Sci USA 1991;88:4646-50.
17. Kajigaya S, Shimada T, Fujita S, Young NS. A genetically engineered cell line that produces empty capsids of B19 (human) parvovirus. Proc Natl Acad Sci USA 1989;86:7601-5.
18. O'Neill HJ, Venugopal K, Coyel PV, et al. Development of an IgM acpture assay for the diagnosis of B19 parvovirus infection using recombinant baculoviruses expressing VP1 or VP2 antigens. Clin Diagn Virol 1995;3:181-90.
19. Cubel RCN, Oliveira SA, Brown DWG, et al. Diagnosis of parvovirus B19 infection by detection of specific immunoglobin M antibody in saliva. J Clin Microbiol 1996;34:205-7.

20. Erdman DD, Usher MJ, Tsou C, et al. Human parvovirus B19 specific IgG, IgA, and IgM antibodies and DNA in serum specimens from persons with erythema infectiosum. J Med Virol 1991;35:110-5.
21. Kurtz JB, Anderson MJ. Cross-reactions in rubella and parvovirus specific IgM tests. Lancet 1985;2:1356.
22. Bruu AL, Nordbø SA. Evaluation of five commercial tests for detection of immunoglobulin M antibodies to human parvovirus B19. J Clin Microbiol 1995;33:1363-5.
23. Söderlund M, Brown CS, Cohen BJ, et al. Accurate serodiagnosis of B19 parvovirus infections by measurement of IgG avidity. J Infect Dis 1995;171:710-3.
24. Koch WC, Massey G, Russell CE, Adler SP. Manifestations and treatment of human parvovirus B19 infection in immunocompromised patients. J Pediatr 1990;116:355-9.
25. Sevall JS. Detection of parvovirus B19 by dot-blot and polymerase chain reaction. Mol Cell Probes 1990;4:237-46.
26. Koch WC, Adler SP. Detection of human parvovirus B19 DNA by using the polymerase chain reaction. J Clin Microbiol 1990;28:65-9.
27. Török TJ, Wang Q-Y, Gary GW, Yang C-F, Finch TM, Anderson LJ. Prenatal diagnosis of intrauterine parvovirus B19 by the polymerase chain reaction technique. Clin Infect Dis 1992;14:149-55.
28. Cohen B, Millar A, Schwind P. Screening blood donations for parvovirus B19. Lancet 1995;346:1631.
29. Harris JW. Parvovirus B19 for the hematologist. Am J Hematol 1992;39:119-30.

Respiratory Syncytial Virus

Pamela Bean, Ph.D.

Respiratory syncytial virus (RSV) causes about 70% of cases of bronchiolitis, which is the single commonest cause of infant hospitalization in the western world.[1] Detection of respiratory syncytial virus (RSV)-specific IgG, IgM and IgA by EIA has overall sensitivity and specificity of 87% and 79%, respectively, with paired acute and convalescent sera.[2] Some heterologous antibody responses are noted with primary and recurrent infections with groups A and B RSV.[3] Diagnosis of acute RSV infection is best accomplished by antigen detection in nasopharyngeal secretions (NPS) by FA or EIA, which have sensitivities of 85-97% and 88–100%,[4-6] and specificities of 91–≥98% and 87–96%, respectively.[4-6] In general, culture is no longer the test of choice, because efficacious treatment with ribavirin[7] mandates laboratory diagnosis more rapidly than the 4-6 days usually required for RSV culture.[8] Shell vial culture techniques, however, can detect RSV with 100% sensitivity after 40 hours; 4% of specimens negative for RSV antigen by IFA and 11% of EIA-negative specimens test positive by shell vial culture.[9] Nasal lavage as compared with NPS has a PPV of 95.6% and NPV of 92.5% for diagnosis of RSV infection.[10]

PCR detection of RSV RNA in nasopharyngeal aspirates is rapid, 95% sensitive and >97% specific. The ability to distinguish RSV subgroups A & B is now possible by RT-PCR.[11] Microneutralization assays using EIA to measure virus neutralization are useful in identification of optimal intravenous immunoglobulin preparations for passive immunization and are promising for assessment of protective RSV antibody titers.[12] A review of the pathogenesis, diagnosis and therapy of viral pneumonias in children, adults and immunocompromised individuals is available.[13]

REFERENCES
1. Openshaw PJM. Immunopathological mechanisms in respiratory syncytial virus disease. Springer Semin Immunopathol 1995;17:187-201.
2. Meddens MJM, Herbrink P, Lindeman J, van Dijk WC. Serodiagnosis of respiratory syncytial virus (RSV) infection in children as measured by detection of RSV-specific immunoglobulins G, M, and A with enzyme-linked immunosorbent assay. J Clin Microbiol 1990;28:152-5.
3. Muelenaer PM, Henderson FW, Hemming VG, et al. Group-specific serum antibody responses in children with primary and recurrent respiratory syncytial virus infections. J Infect Dis 1991;164:15-21.
4. Takimoto S, Grandien M, Ishida MA, et al. Comparison of enzyme-linked immunosorbent assay, indirect immunofluorescence assay, and virus isolation for detection of respiratory viruses in nasopharyngeal secretions. J Clin Microbiol 1991;29:470-4.

5. Thomas EE, Book LE. Comparison of two rapid methods for detection of respiraory syncytial virus (RSV) (TestPack RSV and Ortho RSV ELISA) with direct immunofluorescence and virus isolation for the diagnosis of pediatric RSV infection. J Clin Microbiol 1991;29:632-5.
6. Siqueira MM, Nascimento JP, Portes SA, Schuy W. Enzyme immunoassay for respiratory syncytial virus: rapid detection in nasopharyngeal secretions and evaluation of isolates representing different RSV subgroups. J Clin Lab Anal 1993;7:130-3.
7. Aylward RB, Burdge DR. Ribavirin therapy of adult respiratory syncytial virus pneumonitis. Arch Intern Med 1991;151:2303-4.
8. Kellogg JA. Culture vs direct antigen assays for detection of microbial pathogens from lower respiratory tract specimens suspected of containing the respiratory syncytial virus. Arch Pathol Lab Med 1991;115:451-8.
9. Smith MC, Creutz C, Huang YT. Detection of respiratory syncytial virus in nasopharyngeal secretions by shell vial techniques. J Clin Microbiol 1991;29:463-5.
10. Balfour-Lynn IM, Girdhar DR, Aitken C. Diagnosing respiratory syncytial virus by nasal lavage. Arch Dis Child 1995;72:58-9.
11. Freymuth F, Eugene G, Vabret A, et al. Detection of respiratory syncytial virus by reverse transcription-PCR and hybridization with a DNA enzyme immunoassay. J Clin Microbiol 1995;33:3352-5.
12. Siber GR, Leszczynski J, Pena-Cruz V, et al. Protective activity of a human respiratory syncytial virus immune globulin prepared from donors screened by microneutralization assay. J Infect Dis 1992;165:456-63.
13. Greenberg SB. Viral pneumonia. Infect Dis Clin North Am 1991;5:603-21.

Rhinoviruses

Kevin J. Reagan, Ph.D.

Although most rhinovirus infections resolve without incident, complications including lower respiratory tract infections, pulmonary disease in the immunocompromised and exacerbation of bronchitis and asthma in children indicate the potential for serious illness.[1,2] Rhinoviruses are present in 17% of acute otitis media and are the sole pathogen in 6%.[3] Clinical symptoms make differentiation of rhinovirus versus respiratory syncytial virus or coronavirus infection very difficult.[4] The number of rhinovirus serotypes is near 100 and counting - - making it difficult to ascribe specific characteristics and time frames to all the known rhinoviruses on the basis of the few types studied. Nonetheless, findings based on studies with human rhinovirus 2 (HRV-2) suggest that: 1) virus excretion generally occurs during the period 2-10 days after infection but continues for 16 days in some subjects; 2) asymptomatic subjects may excrete virus; subjects whose symptoms have resolved can remain infectious and continue to excrete virus; 3) HRV-2-specific immunoglobulins in sera and nasal secretions do not increase until 1-2 weeks after inoculation (clinical symptoms appear ~48 hours after inoculation, peak on days 3–4 and generally resolve in 7–10 days); 4) HRV-2 antibodies reach maximum levels 35 days after inoculation; 5) serum neutralizing antibodies remain elevated for many years after infection but local specific antibodies are no longer detectable after 2 years; 6) the pre-inoculation levels of IgA in nasal washings are lower in those who become infected (both asymptomatic and those with colds) than in those who do not; this correlation is again evidenced at reinoculation 1 year later.[5,6] Aspirin and acetaminophen can actually suppress serum antibody responses and lead to increased nasal symptoms and duration of viral shedding.[7] In contrast to virus isolation, EIA is a simple and rapid means of diagnosing rhinovirus infections, but is limited in utility due to cross-reactivity among HRV serotypes. PCR amplification is useful for both for diagnosis and study of rhinoviruses.[8,9] The limited advances in treatment of rhinovirus infection was recently reviewed.

REFERENCES
1. Al-Nakib W, Dearden DJ, Tyrrell DAJ. Evaluation of a new enzyme-linked immunosorbent assay (ELISA) in the diagnosis of rhinovirus infection. J Med Virol 1989;29:268-72.
2. Arola M, Ziegler T, Ruuskanen O, Mertsola J, Näntö-Salonen K, Halonen P. Rhinovirus in acute otitis media. J Pediatr 1988;113:693-5.
3. Barclay WS, Callow KA, Sergeant M, Al-Nakib W. Evaluation of an enzyme-linked immunosorbent assay that measures rhinovirus-specific antibodies in human sera and nasal secretions. J Med Virol 1988;25:475-82.

4. Barclay WL, Al-Nakib W, Higgins PG, Tyrrell DA. The time course of the humoral immune response to rhinovirus infection. Epidemiol Infect 1989;103:659-69.
5. Dearden CJ, Al-Nakib W. Direct detection of rhinoviruses by an enzyme-linked immunosorbent assay. J Med Virol 1987;23:179-89.
6. Forsyth M, Al-Nakib W, Chadwick P, et al. Rhinovirus detection using probes from the 5' and 3' end of the genome. Arch Virol 1989;107:55-63.
7. Gama RE, Horsnell PR, Hughes P-J, et al. Amplification of rhinovirus specific nucleic acids from clinical samples using the polymerase chain reaction. J Med Virol 1989;28:73-7.
8. Olive DM, Al-Mufti S, Al-Mulla W, et al. Detection and differentiation of picornavriuses in clinical samples following genomic amplification. J Gen Virol 1990;71(Pt 9):2141-7.
9. Marlin SD, Staunton DE, Springer TA, Stratowa C, Somergruber W, Merluzzi VJ. A soluble form of intercellular adhesion molecule-1 inhibits rhinovirus infection. Nature 1990;334:70-2.

Chapter 9
The Neuroimmune Axis

Acute-Phase Reactants (CSF)

Gautam Thor, Ph.D.

Altered concentrations of acute-phase reactants are recognized to be indicative of chronic inflammation, and quantitation by rate nephelometry of C-reactive proteins (CRP) is often indicative of the disease progression and could be cytokine dependent.[1] In order to distinguish between bacterial meningitis (BM) and viral meningitis (VM), concentrations of CRP, α_1-antitrypsin α_1-acid glycoprotein (AAG), α_2 ceruloplasmin and α_2 haptoglobin can be measured in CSF and sera.[2] The increased concentrations of AAG and CRP in BM are useful in distinguishing from VM. These results were substantiated in a separate study;[3] the high levels of CRP (>6 µg/mL) were seen in 21 out of 25 cases of children with pyogenic meningitis.

Studies pertaining to amyloidosis, particularly Alzheimer disease (AD), indicate elevated concentrations of serum amyloid protein in the CSF, probably as a consequence of β amyloid deposition.[4] Elevated ceruloplasmin in the CSF of AD patients is also reported[5] and could be a consequence of oxidative stress.[5] Also, elevated concentrations of α_1-antichymotrypsin in CSF and serum are claimed to be useful markers for monitoring disease progression.[6]

REFERENCES
1. Bull BS, Chien S, Dormandy JA, et al. Laboratory techniques: guidelines on selection of laboratory tests for monitoring the acute phase response. J Clin Pathol 1988;41:1203-12.
2. Paradowski M, Lobos M, Kuydowics J, Krakowiak M, Kubasiewics-Ujma B. Acute phase proteins in serum and cerebrospinal fluid in the course of bacterial meningitis. Clin Biochem 1995;28:459-66.
3. Singh N, Arora S, Kahlon PS. Cerebrospinal fluid C-reactive protein in meningitis. Indian Pediatrics 1995;32:687-8.
4. Hawkins PN, Rossor MN, Gallimore JR, Miller B, Moore EG, Pepys MB. Concentration of serum amyloid P component in the CSF as a possible marker of cerebral amyloid deposits in Alzheimer's disease. Biochim Biophys Res Comm 1994;201:722-6.
5. Loeffler DA, DeMaggio AJ, Juneau PL, et al. Ceruloplasmin is increased in cerebrospinal fluid in Alzheimer's disease but not Parkinson's disease. Alzheimer Dis Assoc Disord 1994;8:190-7.
6. Licastro F, Parnetti L, Morini MC, et al. Acute phase reactant α_1-antichymotrypsin is increased in cerebrospinal fluid and serum of patients with probable Alzheimer disease. Alzheimer Dis Assoc Disord 1995;9:112-8.

Brain Complement

Jeffrey W. Terryberry, B.S.

Normally, the CSF concentrations of complement proteins, both terminal complement complexes and membrane attack complexes, are kept extremely low by the action of complement inhibitors which prevent the transfer of complement proteins across the blood-brain barrier, as well as prevent resting microglia from produing complexes.[1,2] Oligodendrocytes and Schwann cells can directly activate the classical complement pathway by binding C1q. Blocking this activation prevents experimental demyelination.[3] In neurodegeneration, microglia and astrocytes upregulate the expression of various complement components. Astroglioma cells synthesize all components of both the classical and alternative pathways. Microglia produce C6, C7, C8 and C9, fluid-phase regulators, S-protein and clusterin (apo J).[2] Astrocytes synthesize C1, C2, C3, C4, C5, C6, C7, C8, C9, factors B, D, H and I, C1 INH, C4 binding protein, decay accelerating factor, membrane cofactor protein, CD59, clusterin, CR2 and C5αR. Neurons can produce C4, CD59, and CR1.[3] Complement activation in the brain is seen in Pick disease, Alzheimer disease, amyotrophic lateral sclerosis, multiple sclerosis, subarachnoid hemorrhage, ischemic stroke, CNS tumors and CNS infections;[1,2,4-6] whereas, peripheral nervous system complement activation is seen in Guillian-Barré syndrome and chronic inflammatory demyelinating polyradiculoneuropathy.[7] Increased CSF C4d is detected in peripheral neuropathy,[7] while in subarachnoid hemorrhage, the C5b-9 terminal complement complex is elevated.[1] Pick bodies are immunoreactive for the membrane attack complex and clusterin.[8] Alzheimer senile plaques stain for C1q, C3, C4, clusterin, S-protein and protectin (CD59), but not the membrane attack complex.[8-11] Clusterin/apo J is currently being evaluated as a marker for neurodegenerative diseases.[8]

REFERENCES

1. Lindsberg PJ, Öhman J, Lehto T, et al. Complement activation in the central nervous system following blood-brain barrier damage in man. Ann Neurol 1996;40:587-96.
2. Gasque P, Fontaine M, Morgan BP. Complement expression in human brain. Biosynthesis of terminal pathway components and regulators in human glial cells and cell lines. J Immunol 1995;154:4726-33.
3. Singhrao SK, Neal JW, Gasque P, Morgan BP, Newman GR. Role of complement in the aetiology of Pick's disease? J Neuropathol Exp Neurol 1996;55:578-93.
4. Barnum SR. Complement biosynthesis in the central nervous system. Crit Rev Oral Biol Med 1995;6:132-46.
5. Serot JM, Bene MC, Faure GC. Comparative immunohistochemical characteristics of human choroid plexus in vascular and Alzheimer's dementia. Hum Pathol 1994;25:1185-90.
6. Terryberry J, Ahmed A, Lacomis D. complement activation in amyotrophic lateral sclerosis. Submitted, 1997.
7. Koguchi Y, Yamada T, Kuwabara S, Nakajima M, Hirayam K. Increased CSF C4d in demyelinating neuropathy indicates the radicular involvement. Acta Neurol Scand 1995;91:56-61.
8. Yasuhara O, Aimi Y, McGreer EG, McGreer PL. Expression of the complement membrane attack complex and its inhibitors in Pick disease brain. Brain Res 1994;652:346-9.
9. Fischer B, Schmoll H, Riederer P, Bauer J, Platt D, Popa-Wagner A. Complement C1q and C3 mRNA expression in the frontal cortex of Alzheimer's disease. J Mol Med 1995;73:465-71.
10. Afagh A, Cummings BJ, Cribbs DH, Cotman CW, Tenner AJ. Localization and cell association of C1q in Alzheimer's disease brain. Exp Neurol 1996;138:22-32.
11. Veerhuis R, van der Valk P, Janssen I, Zhan SS, Van Nostrand WE, Eikelenboom P. Complement activation in amyloid plaques in Alzheimer's disease brains does not proceed further than C3. Virchows Arch 1995;426:603-10.

Eicosanoids

Jeffrey W. Terryberry, B.S.

Central nervous system (CNS) tissue contains 5- and 12-lipoxygenase (LO) enzymes, and their cysteinyl-leukotriene products which are postulated to play roles in neuroendocrine signaling.[1,2] Elevated eicosanoid concentrations are detected in cases of CNS injury, cerebral ischemia and reperfusion, subarachnoid hemorrhage, epilepsy and hypertension.[1,3,4] Intrathecal histamine and thrombin stimulate CNS 12- and 5-LO activities, respectively. Glutamate and norepinephrine also stimulate the formation of the LO products, 12-hydroperoxyeicosatetraenoic and 12-hydroxyeicosatetraenoic acids, which affect sensory neuron membrane currents.[2,4] LTC_4[1] and PGE_2,[5] produced by astroglial cells can play a pivotal role in vasogenic edema, ischemia and post-hemorrhage vasospasm.[3] Cytochrome P450s in the CNS and periphery are also involved in the arachidonic acid cascade (oxygenase and epoxygenase activities); increased epoxygenase activity is associated with hypertension.[6] Tachykinins and cholinergic agonists induce the expression of prostaglandins and thromboxanes.[7] CNS tumors also demonstrate elevated leukotriene (LTB_4) and PGE_2 concentrations.[4,5]

REFERENCES

1. Winking M, Heldt RM, Simmet T. Thrombin stimulates activation of the cerebral 5-lipoxygenase pathway during blood-brain cell contact. J Cerebral Blood Flow Metab 1995;16:737-45.
2. Abe M, Klein M, Steel DJ, et al. Stereochemistry of the *Aplysia* neuronal 12-lipoxygenase: specific potentiation of FMRFamide action by 12(*S*)-HPETE. Brain Res 1995;683:200-8.
3. Ohtsuki T, Matsumoto M, Hayashi Y, et al. Reperfusion induces 5-lipoxygenase translocation and leukotriene C_4 production in ischemic brain. Am J Physiol 1995;37:H1249-57.
4. Houston MC. Nonsteroidal anti-inflammatory drugs and antihypertensives. Am J Med 1991;90:428-78.
5. Makita K, Falck JR, Capdevila JH. Cytochrome P450, the arachidonic acid cascade, and hypertension: new vistas for an old enzyme system. FASEB J 1996;10:1456-63.
6. Hong J-L, Rodger IW, Lee L-Y. Cigarette smoke-induced bronchoconstriction: cholinergic mechanisms, tachykinins, and cyclooxygenase products. J Appl Physiol 1995;78:2260-6.
7. Appleton I, Tomlinson A, Willoughby DA. Induction of cyclo-oxygenase and nitric oxide synthase in inflammation. Adv Pharmacol 1996;35:27-78.

Glucocorticoids and Neurosteroids

Jeffrey W. Terryberry, B.S.

Glucocorticosteroids (GC) are the most potent and effective agents in controlling chronic inflammatory diseases. GCs exert their effects by binding to the cytoplasmic GC receptor which regulates transcription of cytokine genes involved in the inflammatory process.[1,2] The inactivated GC receptor is bound by heat shock protein 90, immunophilin, and other regulatory components.[1] GCs are derived from the hypothalamic-pituitary-adrenal axis (HPA); adrenocorticotropin (ACTH) induces immunosuppressive GC expression.[3,4] GCs regulate the expression of cytokines TNF-α, GC-CSF, IL-1, IL-2, IL-3, IL-4, IL-5, IL-6 and IL-8; whereas, IL-1, IL-6, and TNF-α stimulate the release of GCs in a prostaglandin- and corticotropin-releasing hormone-dependent manner from the HPA. This neuroimmune feedback mechanism associates physiologic stress with inflammation[1-3] and also involves GC regulation of neuropeptides.[5] GCs can also potently inhibit the induction of nitric oxide synthase and stimulate the expression of the 37 kd immunomodulator, lipocortin-1 in PMNL and macrophages. Lipocortin is a potent inhibitor of phospholipase A_2 which releases arachidonic acid for proinflammatory eicosanoid synthesis.[2,6] In addition, GCs upregulate the expression of IL-1 decoy receptor as well as endonucleases involved in eosinophil apoptosis, and downregulate the expression of the eosinophil chemokine, RANTES.[2,7] Endogenous GCs (corticosterone) inhibit the chemotaxis of neutrophils in inflammatory cholestasis.[8] Leukocyte CD18 and endothelial cell ICAM-1 expression are negatively regulated by GCs which reduce neutrophil extravasation.[2,9] GCs also induce a prolonged elevation in plasma cortisol, most of which is bound by corticosteroid binding globulin (CBG). Inflammation and burn injuries reduce CBG levels thereby increasing free cortisol concentrations for activity at wound sites and the immune system.[10] In endotoxemia, GCs reduce pituitary and macrophage expression of the chemokine, migration inhibitory factor.[11]

Inhaled GC therapy is the most effective treatment for asthmatics,[1] and the exogenous GCs, dexamethasone, prednisolone, betamethasone-17-valerate and RU-486 have been used to treat many chronic inflammatory and autoimmune diseases including arthritis, encephalitis, and neurogenic edemas.[2,3,8,9,12]

Studies also show that other neuroactive steroids, such as testosterone, inhibit immunoglobulin production in B cells.[13] Estrogens and dehydroeprandrosterone affect gerontologic pathologies including coronary heart disease, dementia, osteoporosis, cancer and venous thrombosis.[14-17] Estradiol exerts a neuroprotective affect on hippocampal cell and neuroblastoma cell cultures.[18] An additional lipidic component of the neuroimmune axis involves ganglioside and phospholipid signal cascades which modulate lymphocyte cytokine activities.[19,20]

REFERENCES

1. Barnes PJ, Adcock I. Anti-inflammatory actions of steroids: molecular mechanisms. Trends Pharmacol Sci 1993;14:436-41.
2. Barnes PJ. Anti-inflammatory mechanisms of glucocorticoids. Biochem Soc Trans 1995;23:940-5.
3. Kapcala LP, Chautard T, Eskay RL. The protective role of the hypothalamic-pituitary-adrenal axis against lethality produced by immune, infectious, and inflammatory stress. Ann N Y Acad Sci 1995;771:419-37.
4. Chrousos GP. The hypothalamic-pituitary-adrenal axis and immune-mediated inflammation. N Engl J Med 1995;332:1351-62.
5. Karalis K, Mastorakos G, Sano H, Wilder RL, Chrousos GP. Somatostatin may participate in the antiinflammatory actions of glucocorticoids. Endocrinology 1995;136:4133-8.
6. Perretti M, Ahluwalia A, Harris JG, Harris HJ, Wheller SK, Flower RJ. Acute inflammatory response in the mouse: exacerbation by immunoneutralization of lipocortin 1. Br J Pharmacol 1996;117:1145-54.
7. Colotta F, Mantovani A. Induction of the interleukin-1 decoy receptor by glucocorticoids. Trends Pharmacol 1994;15:138-9.
8. Tjandra K, Kubes P, Rioux K, Swain MG. Endogenous glucocorticoids inhibit neutrophil recruitment to inflammatory sites in cholestatic rats. Am J Physiol 1996;270:G821-G825.

9. Farsky SP, Sannomiya P, Garcia-Leme J. Secreted glucocorticoids regulate leukocyte-endothelial interactions in inflammation. A direct vital microscopic study. J Leukoc Biol 1995;57:379-86.

10. Garrel DR. Corticosteroid-binding globulin during inflammation and burn injury: nutritional modulation and clinical implications. Horm Res 1996;45:245-51.

11. Calandra T, Bernhagen J, Metz CN, et al. MIF as a glucocorticoid-induced modulator of cytokine production. Nature 1995;377:68-71.

12. Ahluwalia A, Newbold P, Brain SD, Flower RJ. Topical glucocorticoids inhibit neurogenic inflammation: involvement of lipocortin 1. Eur J Pharmacol 1995;283:193-8.

13. Kanda N, Tsuchida T, Tamaki K. Testosterone inhibits immunoglobulin production by human peripheral blood mononuclear cells. Clin Exp Immunol 1996;106:410-5.

14. Jick H, Derby LE, Myers MW, Vasilakis C, Newton KM. Risk of hospital admission for idiopathic venous thromboembolism among users of postmenopausal oestrogens. Lancet 1996;348:981-3.

15. Tang M-X, Jacobs D, Stern Y, et al. Effect of oestrogen during menopause on risk and age at onset of Alzheimer's disease. Lancet 1996;348:429-32.

16. Barrett-Connor E, Goodman-Gruen D. The epidemiology of DHEAS and cardiovascular disease. Ann N Y Acad Sci 1995;774:259-70.

17. Fishman J, Osborne MP, Telang NT. The role of estrogen in mammary cracinogenesis. Ann N Y Acad Sci 1995;768:91-100.

18. Green PS, Simpkins JW. 17α-estradiol exerts neuroprotective effects on SK-N-SH cells. J Neurosol 1997;17:511-5.

19. Serhan CN, Haeggström JZ, Leslie CC. Lipid mediator networks in cell signaling: update and impact of cytokines. FASEB J 1996;10:1147-58.

20. Ladisch S, Li R, Olson E. Ceramide structure predicts tumor ganglioside immunosuppressive activity. Proc Natl Acad Sci USA 1994;91:1974-8.

Neuropeptides and Other Immunomodulators

Jeffrey W. Terryberry, B.S.

A variety of neuropeptides and hormones are involved in immunomodulation. Those which stimulate polymorphonuclear leukocytes (PMNL)[1] include tachykinins, such as neurokinin A & B, growth hormone, prolactin (PRL), 5-lipoxygenase activating protein, met-enkephalin, thyroid stimulating hormone, insulin, adenocorticotropin releasing hormone (ACTH), corticotropin releasing factor, bombesin, calcitonin gene-related peptide (CGRP), bradykinin, vasoactive intestinal peptide (VIP), thyroxine (T4) and triiodothyronine (T3).[1-8] In contrast, β-endorphin, somatastatin, secretoneurin and melanocyte-stimulating hormone ((MSH) inhibit or deactivate PMNL.[1-8] Leukocyte migration to specific body compartments is regulated by central neuroendocrine pathways, and cytokine production is intrinsically linked to hormone and peptide levels.[1] Prolactin is shown to exerts a synergistic effect with IL-2 in activating lymphokine-activated killer cell cytotoxicity to AIDS-related Burkitt-type lymphomas.[9]

Bombesin-related peptides, which are upregulated in chronic obstructive pulmonary diseases, stimulate alveolar macrophage phagocytosis and the production of superoxide and IL-8 in monocytes.[3] Bradykinin induces the secretion of lipidic and peptidergic chemoattractants for neutrophils, monocytes, and eosinophils. Lipoxygenase inhibitors, leukotriene B4 (LTB4) and PAF, partially inhibit this chemotaxis.[4] Secretoneurin deactivates neutrophil chemotaxis.[5] VIP enhances Ig production via a protein kinase C signal cascade,[10] and neuropeptides modulate the axonal reflex in IgE-mediated skin inflammation.[11]

CGRP and the tachykinins induce neurogenic inflammation and the production of superoxide and nitric oxide.[8,12,13] Local anesthesia, dependent on opioid receptor activation, inhibits SP, CGRP, and NKA-induced neurogenic inflammation.[13,14] Activation of γ opioid receptors by met-enkephalin stimulates polymorphonuclear neutrophils and increases the production of superoxide in the respiratory burst.[15,16] In contrast, μ opioid receptor activation by β-endorphin inhibits neutrophil activation.[1] α-MSH also inhibits neurogenic inflammation induced by IL-1β, IL-6, TNF-α and LTB4.[17]

REFERENCES

1. Šterzl I. Neuroendocrine-immune systems: interactions and regulation. Folio Biologia (Praha) 1996;42:67-9.

2. Kliesch WF, Cruse JM, Lewis RE, Bishop GR, Brackin B, Lampton JA. Restoration of depressed immune function in spinal cord injury patients receiving rehabilitation therapy. Paraplegia 1996;34:82-90.

3. Meloni F, Ballabio P, Bianchi L, Mangiarotti P, Grassi G, Bignamini A, Grassi GG. Bombesin enhances monocyte and macrophage activities: possible role in the modulation of local pulmonary defenses in chronic bronchitis. Respiration 1996;63:28-34.

4. Sato E, Koyama S, Nomura H, Kubo K, Sekiguchi M. Bradykinin stimulates alveolar macrophages to release neutrophil, monocyte, and eosinophil chemotactic activity. J Immunol 1996;157:3122-9.

5. Schratzberger P, Reinisch N, Kähler CM, Wiedermann CJ. Deactivation of chemotaxis of human neutrophils by priming with secretogranin II-derived secretoneurin. Regul Pept 1996;63:65-71.

6. Metwali A, Blum AM, Ferraris L, Klein JS, Fiocchi C, Weinstock JV. Eosinophils within the healthy or inflamed human intestine produce substance P and vasoactive intestinal peptide. J Neuroimmunol 1994;52:69-78.

7. Lammers C-H, Schweitzer P, Facchinetti P, et al. Arachidonate 5-lipoxygenase and its activating protein: prominent hippocampal expression and role in somatostatin signaling. J Neurochem 1996;147:52.

8. Germonpré PR, Joos GF, Everaert E, Kips JC, Pauwels RA. Characterization of neurogenic inflammation in the airways of two highly inbred rat strains. Am J Respir Crit Care Med 1995;152:1796-1804.

9. Gaidano G, Contarini M, Pastore C, Saglio G, Matera L. AIDS-related Burkitt's-type lymphomas are a target for lymphokine-activated killers induced by interleukin-2 and prolactin. Proc Soc Exp Biol Med 1996;213:196-205.

10. Kimata H, Yoshida A, Ishioka C, Fujimoto M, Furusho K. Vasoactive intestinal peptide enhances immunoglobulin production and growth in human plasma cells via mechanisms that may involve protein kinase C. J Clin Endocrinol Metab 1996;81:3024-32.

11. Miller GW, Liuzzi FJ, Ratzlaff RE. Involvement of an axonal reflex in IgE-mediated inflammation in mouse skin. J Neuroimmunol 1995;57:137-41.

12. Kajekar R, Moore PK, Brain SD. Essential role for nitric oxide in neurogenic inflammation in rat cutaneous microcirculation. Evidence for an endothelium-independent mechanism. Circ Res 1995;76:441-7.

13. Donaldson LF, McQueen DS, Seckl JR. Local anaesthesia prevents acute inflammatory changes in neuropeptide messenger RNA expression in rat dorsal root ganglia neurons. Neurosci Lett 1994;175:111-3.

14. Bellibas SE. The effect of human calcitonin gene-related peptide on eosinopil chemotaxis in the rat airway. Peptides 1996;17:563-4.

15. Haberstock H, Marotti T. The relevance of intact enkephalin molecule in predominantly δ opioid receptor mediated superoxide anion release. Neuropeptides 1995;29:357-65.

16. Haberstock H, Marotti T, Banfic H. Neutrophil signal transduction in met-enkephalin modulated superoxide anion release. Neuropeptides 1996;30:193-201.

17. Ceriani G, Macaluso A, Catania A, Lipton JM. Central neurogenic antiinflammatory action of α-MSH: modulation of peripheral inflammation induced by cytokines and other mediators of inflammation. Neuroendocrinology 1994;59:138-43.

Serotonin

Jeffrey W. Terryberry, B.S.

The neurotransmitter, serotonin (5-hydroxytryptamine, 5-HT) is involved in proximal inflammatory signaling through its regulation of vascular tone and expression of proinflammatory neuropeptides and other mediators. Thrombin releases platelet 5-HT and mast cell histamine, causing vasodilation. The 5-HT/histamine H2 receptor antagonist, cyproheptadine, reduces edema formation. The 5-HT antagonist, MCI-9042 reduces changes in platelet morphology following activation by PAF, and decreases platelet aggregation,[1-3] while nitric oxide antagonizes 5-HT-mediated edema and platelet aggregation.[4] Allergens can increase bronchial responsiveness to serotonin, which is IL-4 dependent, indicating that IgE-independent pathways for hypersensitivity reactions exist in mice.[5] Reduced platelet 5-HT and increased urinary 5-hydroxyindoleacetic acid metabolite are detected in migraine patients which can be treated with 5-HT antagonists.[6-8] Elevated 5-HT-induced intracellular calcium is seen in platelets of patients with depression and hypertension,[9] and abnormal platelet uptake of 5-HT is seen in women with Alzheimer disease.[10]

REFERENCES

1. Cirino G, Cicala C, Bucci MR, Sorrentino L, Maraganore JM, Stone SR. Thrombin functions as an inflammatory mediator through activation of its receptor. J Exp Med 1996;183:821-7.
2. Smith CCT. Evidence for separate serotonin and catecholamine compartments in human platelets. Biochim Biophys Acta 1996;1291:1-4.
3. Sanderson HM, Heptinstall S, Vickers J, Lösche W. Studies on the effects of agonists and antagonists on platelet shape change and platelet aggregation in whole blood. Blood Coagul Fibrinolysis 1996;7:245-8.
4. Giraldelo CMM, Zappellini A, Muscará MN, et al. Effect of arginine analogues on rat hind paw oedema and mast cell activation in vitro. Eur J Pharmacol 1994;257:87-93.
5. Brusselle G, Kips J, Joos G, Bluethmann H, Pauwels R. Allergen-induced airway inflammation and bronchial responsiveness in wild-type and interleukin-4-deficient mice. Am J Respir Cell Mol Biol 1995;12:254-9.
6. Jones AL, Roberts RC, Colvin DW, Rubin GL, Coughtrie MWH. Reduced platelet phenolsulphotransferase activity towards dopamine and 5-hydroxytryptamine in migraine. Eur J Clin Pharmacol 1995;49:109-14.
7. Marukawa H, Shimomura T, Takahashi K. Salivary substance P, 5-hydroxytrptamine, and gamma-aminobutyric acid levels in migraine and tension-type headache. Headache 1996;36:100-4.
8. Launay JM, Callebert J, Bondoux D, Loric S, Maroteaux L. Serotonin receptors and therapeutics. Cell Mol Biol 1994;40:327-36.
9. Konopka LM, Cooper R, Crayton JW. Serotonin-induced increases in platelet cytosolic calcium concentration in depressed, schizophrenic, and subsance abuse patients. Biol Psychiatry 1996;39:708-13.
10. Kumar AM, Kumar M, Sevush S, Ruiz J, Eisdorfer C. Serotonin uptake and its kinetics in platelets of women with Alzheimer's disease. Psychiatry Res 1995;59:145-50.

Substance P

Jeffrey W. Terryberry, B.S.

The tachykinin, substance P (SP), a major constituent of the neuroimmune axis and axon reflex, is a main mediator of neurogenic inflammation, inducing vasodilatation and plasma extravasation.[1-4] SP exerts pleiotropic effects which include: release of histamine from mast cells, lymphocyte proliferation, immunoglobulin and cytokine secretion from B cells and monocytes, respectively, macrophage stimulation, immune complex formation, eosinophil peroxidase secretion and chemotaxis in response to platelet activating factor (PAF).[1,5,6] On polymorphonuclear leukocytes (PMNL), SP induces chemotaxis, phagocytosis, respiratory burst activity, exocytosis and antibody-mediated cell cytotoxicity. SP increases superoxide production in PMNL and enhances tumor necrosis factor-dependent interleukin 8 secretion.[1] Primary afferent nerve-derived SP has a proinflammatory effect on neutrophils, resulting in increased adhesion to bronchial epithelial cells in acute and chronic bronchitis.[7] SP levels are elevated in sputum in patients with asthma and chronic bronchitis,[8] as well as nasal allergy.[9] SP induces PMNL infiltration into skin during allergic contact dermatitis.[10]

SP also enhances antigen-evoked mediator release from human nasal mucosa and skin mast cells. These mediators include prostaglandin D2 and leukotriene C4. During the allergic reaction, SP interacts with mast cells to enhance the response to allergen challenge.[2] In allergic rhinitis, SP causes the recruitment of eosinophils after repeated allergen exposure.[11] Eosinophil accumulation (but not SP-induced edema or neutrophil accumulation), is inhibitable by a lipoxygenase inhibitor.[12]

In the vasculature, SP induces intercellular adhesion molecule-1 (ICAM-1) expression on vascular endothelial cells, stimulates mast cell degranulation, and promotes neutrophil transendothelial migration.[13] Eosinophils of inflamed human intestine in ulcerative colitis and Crohn disease produce SP and vasoactive intestinal peptide.[14,15]

HIV infection alters SP immunoregulation of lymphocyte proliferation.[16] SP also modulates the replicative activity of HIV in macrophages.[17] Stress-induced abortion is mediated by SP and prevented by CD8+ T cells.[18]

REFERENCES

1. Serra MC, Calzetti F, Ceska M, Cassatella MA. Effect of substance P on superoxide anion and IL-8 production by human PMNL. Immunology 1994;82:63-9.
2. Baumgarten CR, Witzel A, Kleine-Tebbe J, Kunkel G. Substance P enhances antigen-evoked mediator release from human nasal mucosa. Peptides 1996;17:25-30.
3. Meggs WJ. Neurogenic switching: a hypothesis for a mechanism for shifting the site of inflammation in allergy and chemical sensitivity. Environ Health Perspect 1995;103:54-6.
4. Geppetti P, Bertrand C, Ricciardolo FML, Nadel JA. New aspects on the role of kinins in neurogenic inflammation. Can J Physiol Pharmacol 1995;73:843-7.
5. Bozic CR, Lu B, Höpken UE, Gerard C, Gerard NP. Neurogenic amplification of immune complex inflammation. Science 1996;273:1722-5.
6. Pascual DW, Beagley KW, Kiyono H, McGhee JR. Substance P promotes Peyer's patch and splenic B cell differentiation. In: Mestecky J, et al., editors. Advances in Mucosal Immunology. New York: Plenum Press, 1995:55-9.
7. DeRose V, Robbins RA, Snider RM, et al. Substance P increases neutrophil adhesion to bronchial epithelial cells. J Immunol 1994;152:1339-46.
8. Tomaki M, Ichinose M, Miura M, et al. Elevated substance P content in induced sputum from patients with asthma and patients with chronic bronchitis. Am J Respir Crit Care Med 1995;151:613-7.
9. Konno A, Numata T, Terada N, Hanazawa T, Nagata H, Motosugi H. Role of substance P in the vascular response of nasal mucosa in nasal allergy. Ann Otol Rhinol Laryngol 1996;105:648-53.
10. Goebeler M, Henseleit U, Roth J, Sorg C. Substance P and calcitonin gene-related peptide modulate leukocyte infiltration to mouse skin during allergic contact dermatitis. Arch Dermatol Res 1994;286:341-6.
11. Fajac I, Braunstein G, Ickovic M-R, Lacronique J, Frossard N. Selective recruitment of eosinophils by substance P after repeated allergen exposure in allergic rhinitis. Allergy 1995;50:970-5.
12. Walsh DT, Weg VB, Williams TJ, Nourshargh S. Substance P-induced inflammatory responses in guinea-pig skin: the effect of specific NK_1 receptor antagonists and the role of endogenous mediators. Br J Pharmacol 1995;114:1343-50.
13. Nakagawa N, Sano H, Iwamoto I. Substance P induces the expression of intercellular adhesion molecule-1 on vascular endothelial cells and enhances neutrophil transendothelial migration. Peptides 1995;16:721-5.
14. Metwali A, Blum AM, Ferraris L, Klein JS, Fiocchi C, Weinstock JV. Eosinophils within the healthy or inflamed human intestine produce substance P and vasoactive intestinal peptide. J Neuroimmunol 1994;52:69-78.
15. Suzuki H, Miura S, Liu YY, Tsuchiya M, Ishii H. Substance P induces degranulation of mast cells and leukocyte adhesion to venular endothelium. Peptides 1995;16:1447-52.
16. Covas MJ, Pinto La, Victorino MM. Disturbed immunoregulatory properties of the neuropeptide substance P on lymphocyte proliferation in HIV infection. Clin Exp Immunol 1994;96:384-8.
17. Ho W-Z, Cnaan A, Li Y-H, et al. Substance P modulates human immunodeficiency virus replication in human peripheral blood monocyte-derived macrophages. AIDS Res Hum Retroviruses 1996;12:195-8.
18. Arck PC, Merali F, Chaouat G, Clark DA. Inhibition of immunoprotective CD8[+] T cells as a basis for stress-triggered substance P-mediated abortion in mice. Cell Immunol 1996;171:226-30.

Appendix

Diagnostic Efficiency and Accuracy

Receiver Operating Characteristic Curves

Pamela Bean, Ph.D.

The curve generated by plotting the false-positive rate of a test (one minus the specificity) versus the true-positive rate (sensitivity) for different cut-off values is called the receiver operating characteristic (ROC) curve.[1] This graphic representation of the sensitivity and specificity of a test at various cut-off values provides a means for comparing the accuracy of one test with that of another. The ROC curve visually demonstrates the trade-off between true-positive and false-positive results and identifies the best cut-off value for a test to discriminate between disease and nondisease.[2]

The shape and position of the curved line conveys information about the value of the test. Curves that lie in the upper left-hand corner indicate more accurate tests than those that fall closer to the diagonal.[3] For low-prevalence disorders (in which positive test results are more likely to represent false-positives) or situations in which false-positive results expose the patient to potentially dangerous further testing or treatment, the decision maker should choose a cut-off criterion corresponding to points in the lower left-hand portion of the curve to minimize the number of false-positive results at the expense of more false-negatives. Alternatively, for high prevalence conditions or situations in which the decision maker desires to minimize false-negatives (as in screening for some cancers), a cut-off value should be selected that coincides with points in the plot's upper right-hand portion.[3,4] The area under the ROC curve is a measure of accuracy. If the area beneath the curve is 0.5 or less of the area of the entire graph, then no discrimination exists because such a result can be achieved by chance alone; but if the proportion of the area under the curve is equal to that of the entire graph, then perfect discrimination exits. In the case of perfect discrimination, the curve lies along the upper Y axis and along the top of the graph.[5] An ROC curve useful for summarizing a body of diagnostic accuracy literature, comparing technologies, detecting outliers, and finding the optimum operating point of a test is described as a new tool for technology assessment.[5]

REFERENCES
1. Zweig MH, Campbell G. Receiver-operating characteristic (ROC) plots: a fundamental evaluation tool in clinical medicine [Review]. Clin Chem 1993;39:561-77.
2. Rainer RO, Geisinger KR. Beyond sensitivity and specificity [Editorial]. Am J Clin Pathol 1995;103:541-2.
3. Hagen MD. Test characteristics. How good is that test? Prim Care 1995;22:213-33.
4. Schoonjans F, Depuydt C, Comhaire F. Presentation of receiver-operating characteristic (ROC) plots [Letter]. Clin Chem 1996;42:986-7.
5. Gambino R. The misuse of predictive value - or why you must consider the odds. Ann Ist Super Sanità 1991;27:395-400.
6. Littenberg B, Moses LE. Estimating diagnostic accuracy from multiple conflicting reports: new meta-analytic method. Med Decis Making 1993;13:313-21.

Sensitivity, Specificity and Predictive Values

Pamela Bean, Ph.D.

Sensitivity and specificity provide estimates of how well a particular procedure identifies patients with and without disease, respectively.[1] Sensitivity is the percentage of diseased individuals (as determined by some other gold standard procedure) who have a positive test result. This value, also called the true-positive rate, provides information about those diseased individuals who will not be detected by the procedure but who, rather, demonstrate false-negative results. The false-negative rate is one minus the sensitivity.[2]

Test specificity defines how many normal individuals the test will correctly identify as normal.[1] Specificity, therefore, also describes the true-negative rate for a particular test.

Normal individuals who demonstrate a positive rather that a negative result are false-positives. The false-positive rate and the specificity are complementary values; the false-positive rate is a one minus the specificity.[2] Efficiency is the percentage of test results that are true-positive and true-negative.[3]

Sensitivity and specificity answer the questions: "If the patient has the disease, how likely is he/she to have a positive test?" and "If the patient does not have the disease, how likely is he/she to have a negative test?" The clinician's questions are different: "If the patient has a positive test, how likely is he/she to have the disease?" and "If the patient has a negative test, how likely is he/she not to have the disease?" These indices, the positive predictive value (PPV) and negative predictive value (NPV), respectively, depend not only on sensitivity and specificity but also on the prevalence of the disease.[4,5] A high PPV indicates a strong likelihood that a person with a positive test result has the disease. A high NPV means that a negative result virtually rules out the disease. PV are necessarily approximations and are best based on data derived from tests for which an optimal cut-off point is assigned.[1-7] Predictive value is based on an absolute determination of positive versus negative results; determination of the likelihood of disease considers the strength of the test signal (e.g., high titer, strong positive) and data from confirmatory tests.[8] In all cases involving assessment of the diagnostic value of a test, special attention must be given to potential problems arising from an unrepresentative size or spectrum of the patient sample or from possible selection bias in associating the test result with the disease.[9,10]

Prevalence is the number of patients per 100,000 population who have the disease at a given time.[3]

Incidence derives from *incident* or *event* and is always associated with a stated period of time. The incidence for a disease is the number of patients per 100,000 population who develop the disease in a given year.[3] A chronic disease can have low incidence but high prevalence.[3] The incidence of an acute disease can be high but its prevalence quite low.

$$prevalence = incidence \times duration\ of\ disease^3$$

REFERENCES
1. Hagen MD. Test characteristics. How good is that test? Prim Care 1995;22:213-33.
2. Douglass CW. Evaluating diagnostic tests. Adv Dent Res 1993;7:66-9.
3. Galen RS, Gambino SR, editors. Beyond Normality: The Predictive Value and Efficiency of Medical Diagnoses. New York: John Wiley & Sons, 1975.
4. Rainer RO, Geisinger KR. Beyond sensitivity and specificity [Editorial]. Am J Clin Pathol 1995;103:541-2.
5. Daniel BL, Daniel TM. Graphic representation of numerically calculated predictive values: an easily comprehended method of evaluating diagnostic tests. Med Decis Making 1993;13:355-8.
6. Methods for Prognosis and Decision Making Working Group. Memorandum for the evaluation of diagnostic measures. J Clin Chem Clin Biochem 1990;28:873-9.
7. Reid MC, Lachs MS, Feinstein AR. Use of methodological standards in diagnostic test research. JAMA 1995;274:645-51.
8. Gambino R. The misuse of predictive value - or why you must consider the odds. Ann 1st Super Sanita 1991;27:395-400.
9. Diamond GA. Off Bayes: effect of verification bias on posterior probabilities calculated using Bayes' theorem. Med Decis Making 1992;12:22-31.
10. Choi BC. Sensitivity and specificity of a single diagnostic test in the presence of work-up bias. J Clin Epidemiol 1992;45:581-6.

Allergens Which Stimulate T Cells

Emmanuel A. Ojo-Amaize, Ph.D.

Allergen	T cell Subset	Cytokine Profile
Cryptomeria japonica[1] (Japanese cedar)	$CD4^+/T_H2$	IL-4, IL-5, IL-10
House-dust mite[2]	$CD4^+/T_H2$	IL-4, IL-5, IL-10
House-dust mite (p28-40 analogues with alanine residues at positions 34 and 35)[3]	$CD4^+/T_H1$	IFN-γ
American cockroach C_r-PI allergen[4]	$CD4^+/T_H2$	IL-4
Rye grass (*Lolium perenne*) pollen[5]	$CD3^+$, $CD4^+$	?
Kentucky Bluegrass pollen[6]	$CD4^+/T_H2$	IL-4
Chemicals:[7] Dinitrofluorobenzene (DNFB) Toluene diisocyanate (TDI)	$CD4^+/T_H1$ $CD4^+/T_H2$	IFN-γ IL-4, IL-10
Hen egg[8]	$CD4^+/T_H2$	IL-4, IL-5
Metals:[9,10-12] Pb^{2+}, Ni^{2+}, Zn^{2+}, Be^{2+}, phenyl-Hg, SiO_2, Au, $HgCl_2$	$CD4^+/T_H1$	IL-2, IFN-γ
Pollution, poor sanitation, animal danders and overcrowding[13]	$CD4^+/T_H2$	IL-4, IL-5, IL-6, IL-10, IL-13

REFERENCES

1. Hori T, Kamikawaji N, Kimura A, et al. Japanese cedar pollinosis and HLA-DP5. Tissue Antigens 1996;47:485-91.
2. Ochi H, Tanaka T, Katada Y, et al. Peripheral blood T lymphocytes and basophils, freshly isolated from house-dust-mite-sensitive patients, produce interleukin-4 in response to allergen-specific stimulation. Int Arch Allergy Immunol 1996;111:253-61.
3. Tsitoura DC, Verhoef A, Gelder CM, et al. Altered T cell ligands derived from a major house dust mite allergen enhance IFN-gamma but not IL-4 production by human $CD4^+$ T cells. J Immunol 1996;157:2160-5.
4. Jeng KC, Liu MT, Wu CH, Wong DW, Lan JL. American cockroach C_r-PI allergen induces lymphocyte proliferation and cytokine production in atopic patients. Clin Exp Allergy 1996;26:349-56.
5. Blaher B, Suphioglu C, Knox RB, et al. Identification of T-cell epitopes of Lo1P[9], a major allergen of rye grass (Lolium perenne) pollen. J Allergy Clin Immunol 1996;98:124-32.
6. Zhang L, Yang M, Chong P, Mohapatra SS. Multiple B- and T-cell epitopes on a major allergen of Kentucky Bluegrass pollen. Immunology 1996;87:283-90.
7. Dearman RJ, Basketter DA, Kimber I. Characterization of chemical allergens as a function of divergent cytokine secretion profiles induced in mice. Toxicol Appl Pharmacol 1996;138:308-16.
8. Katsuki T, Shimojo N, Honma K, et al. Establishment and characterization of ovalbumin-specific T cell lines from patients with egg allergy. Int Arch Allergy Immunol 1996;109:344-51.
9. Ojo-Amaize EA, Agopian MS, Peter JB. Novel *in vitro* method for identification of individuals at risk for beryllium hypersensitivity. Clin Diagn Lab Immunol 1994;1:164-71.
10. Ojo-Amaize EA, Conte V, Lin-H-C, et al. Silicone-specific blood lymphocyte response in women with silicone breast implants. Clin Diagn Lab Immunol 1994;1:689-95.
11. Tinkle SS, Kittle LA, Schumacher BA, Newman LS. Beryllium induces IL-2 and IFN-γ in berylliosis. J Immunol 1997;158:518-26.
12. Kiely PD, O'Brien D, Oliveira DB. Anti-CD8 treatment reduces the severity of inflammatory arthritis, but not vasculitis, in mercuric chloride-induced autoimmunity. Clin Exp Immunol 1996;106:280-5.
13. Cookson WOCM, Moffatt MF. Asthma: an epidemic in the absence of infection. Science 1997;275:41-2.

Clusters of Differentiation

Paula D'Amore, Ph.D.

Antigens on the surface of leukocytes are now defined by their reactions with clusters of monoclonal antibodies. Hence, the antigens are referred to as clusters of differentiation (CDs).[1,2]

T Cell Lymphocyte Surface Receptors

CD	Other Names, Function	Cellular Distribution
1a		Thymocytes
1b		Thymocytes
1c		Thymocytes
2	E-rosette receptor Sheep red cell receptor	T cells, NK cells
3	TCR (T cell receptor)	Mature T cells
4		T helper cell subset, Monocytes
5		T cells, B cell subpopulation
7		PAN T cell
8		T cell cytotoxic/ suppressor subpopulation
27		Mature T cells
28	B7/BB1 receptor Activation through binding B7 protein on activated APC (antigen-presenting cells)	T cell subpopulation
38		Activated T-cells, Plasma cells, Thymocytes
45	Leukocyte common antigen (LCA)	Leukocytes
45RA	Isoform of LCA	T-cell subpopulation (naive subset), B cells, Granulocytes, Monocytes
45RO	Restricted T200	T-cell subpopulation (memory cells), Granulocytes, Monocytes

B Cell Lymphocyte Surface Receptors

CD	Other Names, Functions	Cellular Distribution
10	CALLA (Common acute lymphoblastic leukemia antigen)	Lymphoid progenitor cells
19	B4	B lymphocytes
20	B1	B lymphocytes
21	Receptor for Complement fragment	B lymphocyte subpopulation

B Cell Lymphocyte Surface Receptors		
CD	**Other Names, Functions**	**Cellular Distribution**
	C3d (CR2), EBV and CD23	
22		Within cytoplasm - pan B cell marker Surface - B cell subpopulation
23	FcE RII (low affinity FcE receptor)	Activated B cells
24		B cells, Granulocytes
72	(CD5 ligand)	B cells
73	ecto-5'-nucleotidase	B cells, T cell subpopulation
74		B cells
80	B7-1, BB1 ligand for CD28	B cells, Monocytes
81	TAPA-1 (target of an anti-proliferative antibody)	B, T

Myeloid Surface Receptors		
CD	**Other Names, Functions**	**Cellular Distribution**
13		Granulocytes, Monocytes
14		Granulocytes, Monocytes
15		Granulocytes
16	Fcγ RIIIa	Granulocytes, Macrophages, NK cells
32	Fcγ RII	Granulocytes, Monocytes, B cells
33	My 9	Monocytes, Myeloid progenitor cells
34	My 10	Progenitor stem cells, Endothelial cells
35	Receptor for complement fragment C3b/C4b (CR1)	Granulocytes, Monocytes, Some NK cells

NK Cells		
CD	**Other Names, Functions**	**Cellular Distribution**
16	Fcγ RIIIa	NK cells
56	NKH1, N-CAM (neuronal cell adhesion molecule)	NK cells
57	HNK-1	Subset of NK cells
94		NK cells

Adhesion (Integrin) Molecules

CD	Other Names, Functions	Cellular Distribution
11a	LFA-1 α chain, member of the leukocyte cytoadhesion molecule family (CD11a, CD11b, CD11c and CD18)	Most Leukocytes
11b	MAC-1, CR3 (complement C3bi receptor)	Granulocytes, Monocytes, NK cells
11c	Cr4 (complement receptor type 4), α chain of LFA complex	Granulocytes, Monocytes, NK cells
18	LFA-1 β chain	Most Leukocytes Deficiency in CD 18 resulting in decreased expression of CD11a, CD11b, CD11c and CD18 family Leukocyte adhesion deficiency
29	VLA-β chain	Leukocytes
43	Leukosialin, sialophorin (absent in Wiskott Aldrich syndrome)	Leukocytes (except B cells)
44	Hermes antigen, Pgp-I lymphocyte homing, receptor for hyaluronate and proteoglycan	Lymphocytes, Granulocyte, Monocytes
CD49a	VLA-1 α chain associates with CD29-forms VLA-1 (integrin α1 β1) complex Adhesion to collagen, laminin	Activated T and B cells, Endothelial cells
49b	VLA-2 α chain, platelet GP1a. associates with CD29 →VLA-2 (integrin α2β1) complex. Adhesion to collagen	Activated T cells, Platelets
49c	VLA-3 α chain. Associates with CD29→VLA-3 (integrin α3β1). Adhesion to collagen, laminin.	B cells
49c	VLA-4 α chain. Associates with CD29 →VLA-4 (integrin α4β1). Binds fibronectin	Lymphocytes, Monocytes
49e	VLA-5 α chain. associates with CD 29 → VLA-5 (integrin α5β1). Fn receptor	Platelets, Monocytes, Memory T cells

Adhesion (Integrin) Molecules

CD	Other Names, Functions	Cellular Distribution
49f	VLA-6 α chain. associates with CD29 →VLA-6 (integrin α6β1). Laminin receptor.	Platelets
50	ICAM-3 ligand for LFA-1 (CD11a/CD18)	Leukocytes
54	ICAM-1 Primary adhesion ligand for LFA-1 (CD11a/CD18) and CR3 (CD11b/CD18)	Broad
55	DAF (Decay-accelerating factor) Paroxysmal noctural hemoglobinuria (PNH) is caused partially by deficiency of CD55	Broad
58	LFA-3 binds to CD2	Leukocytes
59	(HRF-20) homologous restriction factor PNH-deficiency of CD59	Broad
61	Integrin β3 chain platelet 6PIIIa	Platelets
62E	ELAM-1	Endothelial cells
62L	L-selectin	Broad
62P	PADGEM, P-selectin	Activated platelets
102	ICAM-2 ligand for LFA-1	Lymphocytes, Monocytes, Platelets, Vascular endothelial cells
103	HML-1 (human mucosal lymphocyte-1 antigen)	Mucosal-associated T lymphocytes

Platelets

CD	Other Names, Functions	Cellular Distribution
41	Platelet GPIIb	Platelets
42a	Platelet GPIX	Platelets
42b	Platelet GP1b-x	Platelets
42c	Platelet GP1b-B	Platelets
42d	Platelet GPIV	Platelets
61	Platelet GPIIIa	Platelets

Platelets		
CD	**Other Names, Functions**	**Cellular Distribution**
62P	PADGEM	Activated Platelets
63		Activated Platelets
107a	LAMP1 (Lysosomal-associated membrane protein) expressed on surface of platelet upon activation	Activated Platelets
107b	LAMP2	Activated Platelets

Activation Markers		
CD	**Other Names, Functions**	**Cellular Distribution**
25	IL-2 receptor α chain (TAC)	Activated T, B and Monocytes
26	Dipeptidylpeptidase IV, Ta1	Activated T, B, Macrophages
30	Ki antigen	Activated Lymphocytes Reed-Steinberg cells
69	AIM (activation inducer molecule)	Activated T, B, Monocytes (early activation marker)
70	Ki-24	Activated T, B Reed-Steinberg cells
71	Transferrin receptor	Proliferating T, B, Macrophages
95	APO-1, FAS, member of TNF/NGF family FAS antigen (CD95) and its ligand (Fas L) induce apoptosis	Activated T, Monocytes
96		Activated T

Cytokine Receptors		
CD	**Other Names, Functions**	**Cellular Distribution**
115	CSF-1R (colony-stimulating factor receptor)	Monocytes, Macrophages
w116	GM-CSF (granulocyte-macrophage CSF) receptor	Granulocytes, Monocytes
117	SCF (stem cell factor) receptor, c-kit	Myeloid progenitor cells, Mast cells
w119	Interferon-gamma (IFN-γ) receptor	Monocytes, Granulocytes

Cytokine Receptors		
CD	**Other Names, Functions**	**Cellular Distribution**
120a	TNF (tumor necrosis factor) receptor, 55 kd	Monocytes
120b	TNF receptor, 75 kd	Monocytes, Granulocytes
w121a	IL-1 receptor type I	T cells
w121b	IL-1 receptor type II	Granulocytes
w122	IL-2 receptor B chain	Activated T, NK
w124	IL-4 receptor	T, B
126	IL-6 receptor	Activated B
w127	IL-7 receptor	T cells
w128	IL-8 receptor	Granulocytes

REFERENCES
1. Schlossmann SF, et al. eds. Leukocyte typing V. Vols 1 and 2. Oxford: Oxford University Press, 1995.
2. Stockinger H, Majdic O, Knapp W. 1995 directory for the human leukocyte clusters of differentiation. Transfusion 1996;36:268-305.

Effector Functions of T_H1/T_H2 Subsets of CD4$^+$ T Cells

T Cell Subset	Cytokine Profile	Effector Function
T_H1 Cells	IFN-γ TNF-α TNF-β GM-CSF IL-3	Activation of macrophages leading to microbial killing, cell-mediated immunity and delayed-type hypersensitivity is mediated by IFN-γ.
	IL-2	Expansion of T cells, activation of cytotoxic T lymphocytes and natural killer cells are mediated by IL-2.
T_H2 Cells	IL-4, GM-CSF IL-6 IL-10 IL-3 IL-5 IL-13	IgE production by cells leading to allergies and helminth killing is mediated by IL-4. Eosinophilia leading to helminth killing is mediated by IL-5.

Modified from William OCM, et al. Science 1997;275:41-2.

Factors favoring T_H1 lymphocyte activation include presence of activated CD8$^+$ CTL, adherent cells such as APCs, low antigen dose, antigen requiring phagocytosis and intracellular pathogens. Factors inhibiting T_H1 lymphocyte activation include presence of IL-10 and activated T_H2. Factors favoring T_H2 lymphocyte activation include absence of activated CD8$^+$ CTL, B lymphocytes as APCs, high antigen dose, antigen uptake by pinocytosis and low-dose cyclosporin. Factors inhibiting T_H2 lymphocyte activation include presence of IFN-γ and activation of T_H1 or CD8$^+$ CTL.

Commonly Available RAST Panels

ANIMALS
Cat epithelium
Cow dander
Dog dander
Horse dander

FOODS - NUT MIX
Peanaut
Hazel
Brazil nut
Almond
Coconut

FOODS-SEAFOOD MIX
Fish
Shrimp
Blue mussel
Tuna
Salmon

FOODS - CEREAL MIX
Wheat
Oat
Corn
Sesame seed
Buckwheat

FOODS - CHILDREN'S
FOOD MIX
Egg white
Milk
Wheat
Peanut
Soybean

GRASSES
June-Kentucky Blue
Meadow fescue
Orchard
Perennial rye
Timothy
Bermuda
Johnson

HOUSE DUST
Cockroach
D. farinae
D. pteronyssinus
House dust
  (Hollister-Stier)

MOLDS
Alternaria tenuis
Aspergillus fumigatus
Cladosporium
herbarum
Penicillium notatum

TREES
Birch
Elm
Maple (box elder)
Oak
Walnut

TREES
Cottonwood
Elm
Maple (box elder)
Oak
Pecan pollen

TREES
Cottonwood
Elm
Mesquite
Mountain cedar
Oak

TREES
Cottonwood
Elm
Oak
Sycamore
Willow

TREES
Acacia
Eucalyptus
Olive
White Pine
Willow

WEEDS
Common ragweed
English plantain
Lamb's quarters
Mugwort
Russian thistle

WEEDS
English plantain
Lamb's quarters
Mugwort
Scale
Western ragweed

PEDIATRIC FOOD PANEL
Egg white
Milk
Wheat
Soybean

FOOD PANEL
Egg white
Milk
Codfish
Wheat
Corn
Peas
Peanut
Soybean
Shrimp
Tomato

MOLD PANEL
Penicillium
Cladosporium
Aspergillus
Mucor
Candida
Alternaria tenuis

NORTHEAST PANEL
Timothy grass
June grass
Common ragweed
English plantain
Oak
Cat epithelium
Dog dander
House dust
Mite (*D. farinae*)
Alternaria tenuis

MIDWEST PANEL
Bermuda grass
June/Blue grass
Western ragweed
Mugwort (sage)
Russian thistle
Oak
Elm
Olive
Cat epithelium
Dog dander
Alternaria tenuis
House dust

SOUTHWEST PANEL
Bermuda grass
Perennial rye grass
Mugwort (sage)
Russian thistle
Elm
Cat epithelium
Dog dander
House dust
Mite (*D. farinae*)
Alternaria tenuis

SOUTHEAST PANEL
Bermuda grass
Red top
Common ragweed
English plantain
Oak
Cat epithelium
Dog dander
House dust
Mite (*D. farinae*)
Alternaria tenuis

NORTHERN CALIFORNIA PANEL
Rye grass
June grass
Western ragweed
English plantain
Oak
Cat epithelium
Dog dander
House dust
Mite (*D. farinae*)
Alternaria tenuis

SOUTHERN CALIFORNIA PANEL
Bermuda grass
June grass
Mugwort (sage)
Russian thistle
Oak
Cat
Dog dander
House dust
Mite (*D. farinae*)
Alternaria tenuis

Commonly Available Individual Allergen RAST Tests

DRUGS
ACTH IgE
Chymodactin IgE
Discase IgE
Human insulin IgE
Insulin, Bovine IgE
Insulin, Porcine IgE
Penicilloyl G IgE
Penicilloyl V IgE

EPIDERMALS
Budgerigar droppings IgE
Budgerigar feathers IgE
Budgerigar serum proteins IgE
Canary feathers IgE
Cat epithelium IgE/IgG
Chicken feathers IgE
Cow dander IgE/IgG
Duck feather IgE
Goat epithelium IgE
Goose feathers IgE/IgG
Guinea pig epithelium IgE
Hamster epithelium IgE
Horse dander IgE/IgG
Mixed feathers (chicken, duck, goose) IgE/IgG
Mouse epithelium IgE
Mouse serum proteins IgE
Mouse urine proteins IgE
Parrot droppings IgE
Parrot feathers IgE
Parrot serum proteins IgE
Pig epithelium IgE
Pigeon droppings IgE
Rabbit epithelium IgE
Rat epithelium IgE
Rat serum proteins IgE
Rat urine proteins IgE
Sheep epithelium IgE
Swine epithelium IgE

FOODS
Almond IgE/IgG
Alpha lactalbumin IgE/IgG
American cheese IgE/IgG
Anchovy IgE/IgG
Apple IgE/IgG
Asparagus IgE/IgG

Avocado IgE/IgG
Banana IgE/IgG
Barley IgE/IgG
Beef IgE/IgG
Beet IgE/IgG
Bell pepper IgE/IgG
Beta lactoglobulin IgE/IgG
Black pepper IgE/IgG
Black walnut IgE/IgG
Blueberry IgE/IgG
Blue mussel IgE/IgG
Broccoli IgE/IgG
Buckwheat IgE/IgG
Cabbage IgE/IgG
Cantaloupe IgE/IgG
Carrot IgE/IgG
Casein IgE/IgG
Cashew IgE/IgG
Cauliflower IgE/IgG
Celery IgE/IgG
Cheddar cheese IgE/IgG
Cheese mold type IgE
Chestnut IgE/IgG
Chick pea (garbanzo) IgE/IgG
Chicken IgE/IgG
Chocolate IgE/IgG
Clam IgE/IgG
Cocoa IgE
Coconut IgE/IgG
Codfish IgE
Coffee IgE/IgG
Corn IgE/IgG
Cotton seed IgE/IgG
Crab IgE/IgG
Cucumber IgE/IgG
Dill IgE/IgG
Duck IgE
Eel IgE
Egg white IgE/IgG
Egg (whole) IgE/IgG
Egg yolk IgE/IgG
English walnut IgE/IgG
Flounder IgE/IgG
Garlic IgE/IgG
Goose IgE
Gluten IgE/IgG
Grape IgE/IgG
Grapefruit IgE

Green bean IgE/IgG
Haddock IgE/IgG
Halibut IgE/IgG
Hazel nut IgE/IgG
Herring IgE/IgG
Hops IgE/IgG
Kidney bean IgE/IgG
Kiwi fruit IgE
Lamb IgE/IgG
Lemon IgE
Lentil IgE/IgG
Lettuce IgE/IgG
Lima bean IgE/IgG
Lobster IgE/IgG
Malt IgE/IgG
Mango IgE/IgG
Melons IgE
Milk IgE/IgG
Millet IgE/IgG
Mushroom IgE/IgG
Mussel IgE
Mustard IgE
Mutton IgE
Nutmeg IgE
Oat IgE/IgG
Onion IgE/IgG
Orange IgE/IgG
Oyster IgE/IgG
Parsley IgE
Pea (green) IgE/IgG
Peanut IgE/IgG
Pear IgE/IgG
Pecan IgE/IgG
Perch IgE/IgG
Pineapple IgE/IgG
Pinto bean IgE/IgG
Pork IgE/IgG
Potato IgE/IgG
Psyllium seed IgE/IgG
Red pepper IgE
Rice IgE/IgG
Rye food IgE/IgG
Saccharomyces cerevisiae IgE
Salmon IgE/IgG
Scallops IgE/IgG
Sesame seed IgE/IgG
Shrimp IgE/IgG
Sole IgE/IgG
Soybean IgE/IgG
Spinach IgE/IgG

Spiny lobster IgE
Squash (Summer) IgE/IgG
Strawberry IgE/IgG
Sunflower seed IgE/IgG
Sugarcane IgE/IgG
Sweet chestnut IgE
Sweet potato IgE/IgG
Swiss cheese IgE/IgG
Swordfish IgE/IgG
Tea IgE/IgG
Tomato IgE/IgG
Trout IgE/IgG
Tuna IgE/IgG
Turkey IgE/IgG
Walnut IgE/IgG
Wheat IgE/IgG
White bean IgE
Yeast (baker's) IgE/IgG
Yeast (brewer's) IgE/IgG

GRASSES
Bahia IgE/IgG
Barley IgE
Bermuda IgE/IgG
Brome IgE/IgG
Canary grass reed IgE
Common reed IgE/IgG
Corn IgE
Cultivated oat pollen IgE/IgG
Cultivated rye IgE/IgG
Cultivated wheat pollen IgE/IgG
Johnson IgE/IgG
June-Kentucky blue IgE/IgG
Meadow fescue IgE/IgG
Meadow foxtail IgE/IgG
Orchard IgE/IgG
Perennial rye IgE/IgG
Red top IgE/IgG
Salt grass IgE/IgG
Sweet vernal IgE/IgG
Timothy IgE/IgG
Velvet IgE/IgG
Wild rye IgE

HOUSE DUST
Allergopharma IgE
Bencard IgE
House dust (Greer) IgE
House dust (Greer) IgG
House dust (Hollister-Steir) IgE/IgG

INSECTS
Aedes communis IgE
Ant IgE
Berlin beetle IgE
Blood Worm IgE
Chironomus thummi th. IgE
Cladotanytarsus lewisi IgE
Cockroach IgE
Green nimitti midge IgE
Honeybee venom IgE/IgG
Imported fire ant IgE
Jumper ant IgE
Midge IgE
Mosquito IgE
Paper wasp venom IgE
White-face hornet venom IgE
Yellow hornet venom IgE
Yellow jacket venom IgE/IgG

MITES
Acarus sino IgE
Dermatophagoides farinae IgE/IgG
Dermatophagoides farinae IgE/IgG
Dermatophagoides pteronyssinus IgE/IgG
Glycyphagus domesticus IgE
Storage mite *Acarus* IgE
Storage mite *Lepidoglypus destructor* IgE
Storage mite *Tyrophagus putreus* IgE

MOLDS
Alternaria tenuis IgE/IgG
Aspergillus amstelodami IgE
Aspergillus fumigatus IgE/IgG
Aspergillus versicolor IgE/IgG
Botrytis cinerea IgE
Candida albicans IgE/IgG
Cephalosporium acremonium IgE/IgG
Cladosporium herbarum IgE/IgG
Curvularia lunata IgE
Epicoccum purpurascens IgE
Epidermophyton floccosum IgE/IgG
Fusarium culmorum IgE
Fusarium moniliforme IgE
Helminthosporium halodes IgE/IgG
Mucor racemosus IgE/IgG
Neurospora sitophila IgE
Paecilomyces sp. IgE

Penicillium brevicomp IgE
Penicillium notatum IgE/IgG
Phoma betae IgE/IgG
Pullularia IgE
Rhizopus nigricans IgE
Serpula lacrymans IgE
Sporobolomyces roseus IgE
Stemphylium botrosum IgE
Trichoderma viride IgE/IgG
Trichophyton rubrum IgE/IgG

OCCUPATIONAL
Alpha amylase IgE
Brazilian rubber tree IgE
Castor bean IgE
Chloramine T IgE
Cotton cultivated IgE
Ethylene oxide IgE
Formaldehyde IgE
Green coffee bean IgE
Hop IgE
Isocyanate HDI IgE
Isocyanate MDI IgE
Isocyanate TDI IgE
Ispaghula IgE
Latex IgE
Phthalic anhydride IgE
Sheep's wool IgE
Silk IgE
Silk waste IgE
Trimetallic anhydride IgE

PARASITES
Ascaris IgE
Echinococcus IgE
Schistosoma IgE

TREE POLLENS
Acacia IgE
Alder IgE/IgG
Australian pine IgE/IgG
Bayberry IgE/IgG
Beech IgE/IgG
Black locust IgE/IgG
Birch IgE/IgG
Black walnut IgE/IgG
Chestnut IgE
Cottonwood IgE/IgG
Douglas fir IgE/IgG
Elder IgE

Elm IgE/IgG
Eucalyptus IgE/IgG
Hackberry IgE/IgG
Hazel nut IgE/IgG
Iodine bush IgE/IgG
Italian cypress IgE
Lilac IgE
Lime tree IgE
Live oak IgE/IgG
Loblolly pine IgE/IgG
Maple-box elder IgE/IgG
Melaleuca IgE/IgG
Mesquite IgE/IgG
Mountain cedar IgE/IgG
Olive IgE/IgG
Pecan IgE/IgG
Pepper tree IgE/IgG
Poplar IgE/IgG
Privet IgE/IgG
Queen palm IgE/IgG
Sycamore IgE/IgG
Walnut IgE/IgG
White Ash IgE/IgG
White oak IgE/IgG
White mulberrry IgE
White pine IgE/IgG
White poplar IgE/IgG
Willow IgE/IgG

WEED & FLOWER POLLENS
Burweed IgE/IgG
Camomile IgE
Careless weed IgE
Cocklebur IgE
Colza IgE
Dandelion IgE/IgG
English plantain IgE/IgG
False ragweed IgE/IgG
Geranium IgE
Giant ragweed IgE/IgG
Golden rod IgE/IgG
Grama grass IgE/IgG
Kochia (firebush) IgE/IgG
Lambs quarters IgE/IgG
Marsh elder (Rough) IgE/IgG
Mugwort IgE/IgG
Nettle IgE
Ox-Eye Daisy IgE
Pigweed (Rough) IgE/IgG
Rose IgE

Russian thistle IgE/IgG
Salt grass IgE/IgG
Scale IgE
Sheep Sorrel IgE/IgG
Short ragweed IgE/IgG
Spiny pigweed IgE/IgG
Sunflower IgE/IgG
Tobacco IgE/IgG
Tulip IgE
Western ragweed IgE/IgG
Worm wood IgE/IgG
Yellow dock IgE/IgG

OTHER
Staphylococcus aureus IgE
Seminal fluid

List of Abbreviations

Ab	=	Antibody
Ab Index	=	Antibody Index
ABIF	=	Avidin-biotin immunofluorescence
ACIF	=	Anticomplement Immunofluorescence
AE	=	Agarose Electrophoresis
Ag	=	Antigen
B	=	Biochemical Assay
bcr	=	Breakpoint cluster region
CAE	=	Cellulose Acetate Electrophoresis
CD	=	Clusters of Differentiation
cDNA	=	Complementary DNA
CF	=	Complement Fixation
CIA	=	Chemiluminescence Assays
CIE	=	Counterimmunoelectrophoresis
CoA	=	Coagglutination
CSF	=	Cerebrospinal Fluid
DA	=	Direct Agglutination
DFA	=	Direct Fluorescent Antibody
DIF	=	Direct Immunofluorescence
DOT BLOT	=	DNA Dot-blot Hybridization
EIA	=	Enzyme Immunoassay
ELISA	=	Enzyme-linked Immunosorbent Assay
EMIT	=	Enzyme-multiplied Immunoassay
EP	=	Electrophoresis
F	=	Fluorimetry
FA	=	Fluorescent Antibody
FC	=	Flow Cytometry
FLO	=	Flocculation
FPIA	=	Fluorescence Polarization Immunoassay
H	=	Hemolytic Assay
HA	=	Hemagglutination
HAI or HI	=	Hemagglutination Inhibition
HPLC	=	High Pressure Liquid Chromatography
ICA	=	Immunocytochemical Assay
ID	=	Immunodiffusion (Double Diffusion)
IEF	=	Isoelectricfocusing
IEP	=	Immunoelectrophoresis
IF	=	Immunofluorescence
IFA	=	Indirect Fluorescent Antibody
IFE	=	Immunofixation Electrophoresis
Ifix	=	Immunofixation
IHA	=	Indirect Hemagglutination
Inh EIA	=	Inhibition Enzyme Immunoassay
IP	=	Immunoperoxidase
IRMA	=	Immunoradiometric Assay
kd	=	kilodalton
LM	=	Light Microscopy
LMC	=	Lymphocyte Microcytotoxicity
LA	=	Latex Agglutination
Mab	=	Monoclonal Antibody
MAC	=	IgM Antibody Capture

MAC EIA	=	IgM Antibody Capture EIA
MEIA	=	Microparticle Enzyme Immunoassay
Micro-IF	=	Micro-Immunofluorescence
mRNA	=	Messenger RNA
NB	=	Northern Blot (RNA hybridization)
NEPH	=	Nephelometry
Nt	=	Neutralization
PCR	=	Polymerase Chain Reaction
PEG	=	Polyethylene Glycol
PEP	=	Protein Electrophoresis
RAST	=	Radioallergosorbent Test
REA	=	Radiative Energy Attenuation
RFU	=	Relative Fluorescent Units
RIA	=	Radioimmunoassay
RID	=	Radial Immunodiffusion
RIP	=	Radioimmunoprecipitation
RIPA	=	Radioimmunoprecipitation Assay
rRNA	=	Ribosomal RNA
RT-PCR	=	Reverse Transcriptase PCR
S	=	Spectrophotometry, Ultraviolet or Visible
SB	=	Southern Blot (DNA hybridization)
SD	=	Standard Deviation(s)
SF	=	Synovial Fluid
snRNP	=	Small nuclear ribonucleoproteins
TA	=	Tube Agglutination
TCA	=	Tissue Culture Assay
TDE(2DE)	=	Two-dimensional Electrophoresis
WB	=	Immunoblot/Western Blot

Methodology Guide

1. **SEPARATION ANALYSES**
   EP   Electrophoresis
   FC   Flow Cytometry
2. **SOLUBLE ANTIGEN-ANTIBODY REACTION ASSAYS**
   ID or DD   Immunodiffusion or Double Diffusion
   RID   Radial immunodiffusion
   CIE   Counterimmunoelectrophoresis
   IEP   Immunoelectrophoresis
   IFIX   Immunofixation
3. **PARTICULATE ANTIGEN-ANTIBODY REACTION ASSAYS**
   DA   Direct Agglutination
   HA   Hemagglutination
   LA   Latex Agglutination (Latex Particle Agglutination)
   CoA   Coagglutination
   HI or HAI   Hemagglutination inhibition
   NEPH   Nephelometry
4. **RBC LYTIC ASSAYS FOR DETECTING ANTIGEN-ANTIBODY REACTIONS**
   CF   Complement Fixation
   Nt   Neutralization
5. **IMMUNOHISTOCHEMICAL ASSAYS**
   FA   Fluorescent Antibody
   DFA   Direct Fluorescent Antibody
   IFA   Indirect Fluorescent Antibody
   ACIF   Anticomplement Immunofluorescence
   ABIF   Avidin-biotin immunofluorescence
   Micro-IF   Micro-immunofluorescence
   IP   Immunoperoxidase
   ICA   Immunocytochemical Assay
6. **IMMUNOASSAY PROCEDURES**
   RIA   Radioimmunoassay
   IRMA   Immunoradiometric Assay
   RAST   Radioallergosorbent Test
   FPIA   Fluorescence Polarization Immunoassay
   CIA   Chemiluminescence Assays
   EIA   Enzyme Immunoassay
   EMIT   Enzyme-multiplied Immunoassay
   ELISA   Enzyme-linked Immunosorbent Assay
   MAC   IgM Antibody Capture
   MEIA   Microparticle Enzyme Immunoassay
   RIPA   Radioimmunoprecipitation Assay
7. **TECHNIQUES IN MOLECULAR BIOLOGY**
   DOT BLOT   DNA Dot-blot Hybridization
   PCR   Polymerase Chain Reaction
   RT-PCR   Reverse Transcriptase PCR
   SB   Southern Blot
   NB   Northern blot
   WB   Immunoblot/ Western Blot

SEPARATION ANALYSES

Electrophoresis (EP) is a technique for separation of ionic molecules (principally proteins) by the differential migration through a gel according to the size and ionic charge of the molecules in an electrical field. Smaller molecules with a more negative charge will travel faster and further through the gel toward the anode of an electrophoretic cell when high voltage is applied. Similar molecules will group on the gel. They may be visualized by staining and quantitated, in relative terms, using densitometers which continuously monitor the photometric density of the resulting stain.

Flow cytometry (FC) is an emerging technique which holds great promise for the separation, classification and quantitation of blood cells and antibodies which affect blood cells. Complex computerized instruments are used to pass a monocellular stream of cells, platelets or other microscopic particulate elements through a beam of laser light. The cells are categorized first by size and then computer analyzed to sort the mixture of cellular elements into cell type by size. In addition, monoclonal antibodies to specific cell surface markers are conjugated to fluorescent dyes and each cell displaying appropriate fluorescent light emission is counted. Tabulation of counted data in conjunction with size analysis enables determination of relative percentages of each specific cellular subset for which monoclonal antibody conjugates are utilized, even when the size of the cell is identical to other subset species.

SOLUBLE ANTIGEN-ANTIBODY REACTION ASSAYS

Immunodiffusion (ID), also called **Double diffusion** (DD) or the Ouchterlony technique, is the classical procedure used to detect the presence of antibodies and determine their specificity by visualization of "lines of identity" (precipitin lines). These precipitin lines (precipitated antigen-antibody complexes) form where the binding concentrations of antigen and antibody are equivalent. Patient serum diffuses from one well through the gel and reacts with a known specific antigen (or antibody) which diffuses through the gel from a second well. DD is strictly qualitative, although the density of the precipitin line and the distance of the line from the sample well may give some indication of the antibody concentration.

Radial immunodiffusion (RID) is a quantitative variation of the Ouchterlony technique (immunodiffusion) in which the agar gel contains evenly distributed antigen (or antibody) and its counterpart from the test sample diffuses into the gel from a single well resulting in a circular precipitin line around the sample well. The diameter of the precipitin ring is proportional to the concentration of the antibody (or antigen) present in the test sample. By comparing the diameter of the test specimen precipitin ring to known standards, a relatively insensitive estimation of the concentration of specific antibody or antigen can be achieved.

Counterimmunoelectrophoresis (CIE) is a procedure in which oppositely charged antigen and antibody are propelled toward each other by an electrical field. This reduces the time necessary for visualization of the antigen-antibody reaction from 18-24 hours in ID to less than one hour and also substantially increases the sensitivity of the analysis. CIE has the capability of detecting concentrations of antigen/antibody 10 times smaller than the lowest concentrations measurable by DD or ID.

Immunoelectrophoresis (IEP) is a two-step procedure which first involves the electrophoretic separation of proteins, followed by the linear diffusion of antibodies into the electrophoretic gel from a trough which extends through the length of the gel adjacent to the electrophoretic path. The antigen-antibody reactions produce precipitin arcs at positions where equivalence occurs. Although quantitation is subjective, an experienced eye can determine not only the presence of the antigen but, through visual comparison to normal control sera, may discriminate relative increases or decreases of antigen by gauging the length and density of the precipitin arcs at positions established for specific antigens using known standards.

Immunofixation (IFIX) is a powerful enhancement of immunoelectrophoresis in which a series of post-electrophoretic gel slabs are layered with cellulose-acetate gels saturated with specific antibodies. The resulting antigen-antibody complexes fixed on the second gel may then be stained, allowing sensitive and specific qualitative visual identification of paraproteins by electrophoretic position.

PARTICULATE ANTIGEN-ANTIBODY REACTION ASSAYS

Direct agglutination (DA) is a general term for techniques which use the agglutination (macroscopic clumping) of particulate reagents as an indicator of the presence of an antigen-antibody reaction. Examples (HA, LA and CoA) follow.

Hemagglutination (HA) is a technique for detecting specific antibodies which, when present, will cause antigen-coated reagent erythrocytes to agglutinate. Crude quantitation of the antibodies can be achieved by performing a serial dilution of the patient serum and noting the highest dilution (titer) at which agglutination is still present.

Latex agglutination (LA), also known as latex particle agglutination, for detection of antibodies is identical to HA in principle, but the substitution of smaller, antigen-coated latex particles for erythrocytes results in improved sensitivity and reagent longevity. Alternatively, antibodies can be absorbed to the latex particles (under appropriate ionic and pH conditions) by binding to the Fc region of antibodies, leaving the Fab region free to interact with antigens present in the applied specimens. This phenomenon has made LA a popular technique for detecting antigens as well.

Coagglutination (CoA) is similar to the LA technique for detecting antigen (described above). Protein A, a uniformly distributed cell wall component of *Staphylococcus aureus*, is able to bind to the Fc region of most IgG isotype antibodies leaving the Fab region free to interact with antigens present in the applied specimens. The visible agglutination of the *S. aureus* particles indicates the antigen-antibody reaction.

Hemagglutination inhibition (HI), also abbreviated HAI, is a variation of the HA technique. Some viral antigens, when coated on erythrocytes, spontaneously cause agglutination in the absence of antibody. In these situations, the specific antigen-antibody reaction actually prevents the agglutination of reagent RBCs. HAI cannot differentiate between isotypes of specific antibodies (IgG, IgA or IgM) although positive HAI analysis of specimens treated with *Staphylococcus aureus* Protein A (discussed above under CoA) to remove the IgG isotype antibodies has been used to imply the presence of specific IgM antibodies to the specific viral antigen. The crude quantitation of the specific antibodies is possible using serial dilution (titer).

Nephelometry (NEPH) is used to quantitate antigen by analyzing increases in turbidity, as measured by increasing scatter of laser light. The interaction of specific antibodies in the reagent with the antigen from the sample results in the formation of antigen-antibody complexes which are rendered insoluble by the presence of precipitating reagents. Most modern nephelometers compare the rate of formation of antigen-antibody complexes (determined by computer analysis of laser light scatter data) to that of known antigenic standards in order to measure precisely the protein antigens (some of which are actually immunoglobulins) present in moderate concentrations.

RBC LYTIC ASSAYS FOR DETECTING ANTIGEN-ANTIBODY REACTIONS

Complement fixation (CF) is an exacting, complex yet sensitive procedure that detects the presence of a specific antigen-antibody reaction by causing the *in vitro* activation of complement via the classical pathway. If complement is not fixed, lysis of the pre-antibody-coated reagent erythrocytes occurs. Again, crude quantitation of antibodies is possible by determining the highest dilution (titer) at which lysis does not occur. The differentiation of specific antibody isotype is not possible.

Neutralization (Nt) is similar to complement fixation but is applicable only in certain pathogenic situations where the antibody being measured is directed against a hemolysin (a bacterial toxin capable of directly lysing erythrocytes). In these situations, the hemolysin and reagent erythrocytes are added, and if the antibody to the hemolysin is present, the lysis of RBCs will not occur. As in CF, crude quantitation is afforded by serial dilution which may be quantitatively compared to established standard material dilutions.

IMMUNOHISTOCHEMICAL ASSAYS

Fluorescent antibody (FA) assay is a general term for procedures which utilize the visual detection of fluorescent dyes coupled (conjugated) to antibodies which react with the antigen when present using fluorescent microscopy. FA allows a competent technologist to identify visually the site of the antigen-antibody reaction thereby rendering significant specificity. Variations are further explained below (DFA, IFA, ACIF, ABIF and Micro-IF).

Direct fluorescent antibody (DFA) is the straightforward detection of antigens using fluorescently labeled antigen-specific antibody. Because detection of the antigen in a substrate of patient sample (cellular smear, fluid or patient-inoculated culture medium) is the goal, DFA is seldom quantitative.

Indirect fluorescent antibody (IFA) is the detection of antibodies to specific antigenic material in the substrate using fluorescent microscopy. Using fluorescently conjugated antibodies which are specific for a particular isotype of antibody, it is possible to distinguish IgG, IgA and IgM isotypes of specific antibodies using IFA. This sensitive technique is highly specific in well-trained hands and recent developments in the establishment of internationally recognized standard materials have led to accurate quantitation of antibody concentrations through endpoint titration (the highest serial dilution of specimen at which specific fluorescence remains) and through measuring visual intensity of fluorescence compared to known reference standard material.

Anticomplement immunofluorescence (ACIF) is a technique used to make certain indirect fluorescent antibody techniques more specific and sensitive. Here the fluorescent dye is conjugated to antibody directed at complement and then added to a complement-fixing complex of antigen and patient antibody.

Avidin-biotin immunofluorescence (ABIF) holds promise for more sensitive and specific amplification of indirect fluorescent antibody procedures. Antibody to the patient's specific antibodies is labeled with biotin, a compound capable of specifically binding avidin in high concentrations. Fluorescently labeled avidin is then added and fluorescent microscopy is used to detect the presence of the complexes.

Micro-immunofluorescence (Micro-IF) is really multiple IFA. Several different substrates are arranged in specific locations on a single microscope slide well allowing a rapid, simultaneous IFA on each substrate.

Immunoperoxidase (IP) assays are analogous to IFA in that antibody presence is identified on antigenic substrates visually. However, in the indirect IP instead of fluorescent dye-antibody conjugates, enzyme-antibody conjugates (principally peroxidase enzymes) are reacted with their corresponding substrates to produce a product which can be seen with a light microscope, eliminating the requirement for costly fluorescent microscopic equipment.

Immunocytochemical assay (ICA) involves the computerized assessment of microscopic fields following DFA, IFA or indirect or direct IP analysis of biopsy tissue from the patient. In addition to improved specificity with the removal of operator subjectivity, the quantifiability of results through computer data analysis of color, intensity and concentration has only begun to be realized.

IMMUNOASSAY PROCEDURES

Radioimmunoassay (RIA) uses fixed-dose, low-level, radioactive-isotope-labeled antigen ("tracer") to compete with unlabeled antigen from the patient specimen for a fixed number of antibody binding sites. Traditional RIA is done with specific antibodies in liquid solution. Solid-phase RIA involves the use of antibody bound to solid support (e.g., tubes, glass beads or plastic fins). The amount of antigen in the specimen is determined by comparing the bound radioactivity with a standard curve.

Immunoradiometric assay (IRMA) uses low-level radioactively labeled specific antibody to quantitate low concentration compounds. In IRMA, a first antibody is presented on solid-phase (coated on tubes or beads). After binding the antigen present in the sample, a second radioactively labeled antibody is added. Radioactivity remaining after washing the solid phase is proportional to the concentration of antigen present in the sample and is quantitated by comparison to a standard curve.

Radioallergosorbent test (RAST) is the name given to an *in vitro* technique which detects the presence of IgE (and IgG) antibodies to allergens, proteins which may give rise to hypersensitivity reactions seen in allergies. Allergens are coated on a complex carbohydrate matrix called a sorbent. Antibodies specific for the allergen being tested bind to the allergen and, if present, are detected by a low-level radioactively labeled antibody to either human IgE or IgG, depending upon the isotype being tested.

Fluorescence polarization immunoassay (FPIA) is a technique which takes advantage of the increased polarization (non-random propagation of emission) of fluorescent light emissions when a fluorescently labeled antigen is bound by reagent antibody. The higher the concentration of unlabeled patient antigen present in the test mixture, the less bound fluorescent antigen is present and, consequently, the lower the polarization of the fluorescent light emission. Standard calibration yields quantitative results.

Chemiluminescence assays (CIA), including a subcategory using bioluminescence (biologically derived chemiluminescence agents), use the generation of light from oxidative chemical reactions as an indicator of the quantity of unbound luminescently labeled antigen. This allows quantitation of unlabeled antigen from patient specimens in a variety of homogeneous (single phase) or heterogeneous (multiple phase) immunoassay techniques.

Enzyme immunoassay (EIA) is the general term for an expanding technical arsenal of testing which allows a full range of quantitative analyses for both antigen and antibodies. These tests use color-changed products of enzyme-substrate interaction (or inhibition) to measure the antigen-antibody reaction. Examples of EIA procedures (EMIT, ELISA, MAC, MEIA) follow.

Enzyme multiplied immunoassay technique (EMIT) is a homogeneous (single phase) EIA procedure in which the antigen being measured competes for a limited number of antibody binding sites with enzyme labeled antigen. The reagent antibody has the ability to block enzymatic activity when bound with the reagent enzyme-antigen complex preventing it's formation of product in the presence of substrate. The free antigen-enzyme complexes resulting from competition with measured antigen in the sample forms color-change products proportional to the concentration of antigen present in the specimen.

Enzyme-linked immunosorbent assay (ELISA) is a sensitive, heterogenous (multiple phase) analytical technique for quantitation of antigen or antibody in which enzyme-labeled antibody

156

or antigen is bound to a solid support (e.g., tubes, beads, microtiter plate wells, plastic tines or fins). After addition of patient specimen and substrate, antigen, antibody or complex are detected by a color change indicating the presence of the product of an enzyme-substrate reaction. Direct ELISA is a technique for measuring antigen using competition for antibody binding sites between enzyme-labeled antigen and patient antigen. Indirect ELISA, or enzyme immunometric assay, measures antibody concentrations using bound antigen to interact with specimen antibodies. Enzyme-labeled reagent antibodies can be isotype-specific (i.e., capable of determining the presence of IgG, IgA, IgM or IgE classes which react with the antigen of interest). The specificity of indirect ELISA assays for IgM isotypes in some infectious diseases is limited by false-positive results due to IgM rheumatoid factor in the presence of IgG-specific antibodies.

IgM antibody capture ELISA (MAC ELISA) has been developed to impart significant improvement in assay specificity to indirect ELISA procedures for IgM isotype antibodies. Solid-phase support (usually microtiter plate wells) are coated with anti-human IgM antibodies capable of binding all IgM isotype antibodies present in the specimen. Reagent antigen is then added, followed by enzyme-labeled antigen-specific antibodies. If IgM antibodies specific for the antigen in question are present, the "sandwich" complex will result in enzymatic color-change proportional to the concentration of IgM-specific antibody present. This technique appears to be the method of choice in many highly specific and more sensitive assays for IgM infectious disease antibodies.

Microparticle enzyme immunoassay (MEIA) is a technique in which the solid-phase support consists of very small microparticles in liquid suspension. Specific reagent antibodies are covalently bound to the microparticles. Antigen, if present, is then "sandwiched" between bound antibodies and antigen-specific, enzyme-labeled antibodies. Antigen-antibody complexes are detected and quantitated by analysis of fluorescence from the enzyme-substrate interaction.

Radioimmunoprecipitation assay (RIPA) is the term used to describe the qualitative assay used as a confirmatory procedure for some antibodies to viral antigens. Viral-infected cell cultures are radioactively labeled and lysed to yield radiolabeled antigen fragments. Specific antibodies, if present, will bind these antigen fragments and the resulting antigen-antibody complexes are precipitated using protein A, boiled to free the immune complexes which are then separated by electrophoresis. The pattern of antigenic moieties to which antibodies are present may then be detected using autoradiography (the exposure of sensitive X-ray film by the radioactive emissions of the bound, labeled antigens). Comparison to labeled molecular weight standards electrophoresed in the same run allows determination of the molecular weight "bands" of antigen to which antibodies are present.

TECHNIQUES IN MOLECULAR BIOLOGY
DNA "dot-blot" hybridization (DOT-BLOT) is a rapid technique used to detect the presence of a specific DNA in a specimen. Dots, or spots of the DNA containing sample are placed onto a nitrocellulose membrane and fixed. This membrane is then hybridized to a radioactively labeled DNA segment of known sequence, specific for the pathogenic DNA being tested. If the pathogenic DNA is present in the specimen, complementary DNA sequences present on the membrane will hybridize, or anneal, producing a double-stranded DNA segment with the radioactive label incorporated into the molecule. The presence of radioactivity is detected by autoradiography.

Polymerase chain reaction (PCR) is a highly efficient method to amplify low levels of specific DNA sequences in a sample to reach the threshold of detection. Two short DNA "primers", oligonucleotides (small portions of a single DNA strand) specific for the pathogenic DNA sought whose sequence flanks that section of DNA to be amplified, are used. Repeated cycles of DNA denaturation (separation of the double DNA strands), primer annealing (recombination of the double-stranded structure) and extension of the primed DNA sequence (by the enzyme DNA polymerase in the presence of added purine and pyrimidine bases) are performed. Each cycle doubles the amount of specific DNA sequence present and results in an exponential accumulation of the DNA fragment being amplified. The reaction products are hybridized to a radioactively labeled DNA segment complementary to a short sequence of the amplified DNA. Following electrophoresis, the radiolabeled product of specific size is detected by autoradiography.

Reverse Transcriptase PCR (RT-PCR) is a technique used to amplify RNA targets. The specimen containing the target RNA (e.g., HIV-1 RNA, Hepatitis C Virus RNA) is subjected to reverse transcription to make complementary DNA (cDNA), which is then, in turn, amplified by PCR.

Southern blot (SB) describes the technique first developed by the Scottish molecular biologist Edward M. Southern which now bears his name. Specimen DNA is denatured, treated with restriction enzymes to result in DNA fragments and then the single-stranded DNA fragments are separated by electrophoresis. The electrophoretically separated fragments are then blotted to a nitrocellulose membrane, retaining their electrophoretic position, and hybridized with radiolabeled single-stranded DNA fragments with sequences complementary to those being sought. The resulting double-stranded DNA bearing the radiolabel is then, if present, detected by autoradiography.

Northern blot (NB) uses techniques similar to the Southern blot described above. Messenger-RNA from the specimen is separated by electrophoresis and blotted to a specially modified paper support to result in covalent fixing of the mRNA in the electrophoretic positions. Radiolabeled single-stranded DNA fragments complementary to the specific mRNA being sought are then hybridized to the bound mRNA. If the specific mRNA is present, the radioactivity is detected by autoradiography. The derivation of this technique from the Southern blot used for DNA detection has led to the common usage of the term "Northern blot" for the detection of specific mRNA.

Immunoblot, commonly referred to as "Western blot" (WB) because of the similarity to the procedures described above, is used to detect antibodies to specific epitopes of electrophoretically separated subspecies of antigens. Electrophoresis of antigenic material yields separation of the antigenic components by molecular weight. Blotting of the separated antigen to nitrocellulose, retaining the electrophoretic position, and reacting it with patient specimen will result in the binding of specific antibodies, if present, to each antigenic "band." Electrophoresis of known molecular weight standards allows for the determination of the molecular weight of each antigenic band to which antibodies may be produced. These antibodies are then detected using EIA reactions which characterize antibody specificity. This technique is often used to confirm the specificity of antibodies which are detected by ELISA screening procedures.

Index